Methods in Molecular Biology

Series Editor
John M. Walker
School of Life and Medical Sciences
University of Hertfordshire
Hatfield, Hertfordshire, AL10 9AB, UK

For further volumes:
http://www.springer.com/series/7651

Multiple Myeloma

Methods and Protocols

Edited by

Christoph Heuck

Janssen R&D, Spring House, PA, USA

Niels Weinhold

The Myeloma Institute, University of Arkansas for Medical Science, Little Rock, AR, USA

Humana Press

Editors
Christoph Heuck
Janssen R&D
Spring House, PA, USA

Niels Weinhold
The Myeloma Institute
University of Arkansas for Medical Science
Little Rock, AR, USA

ISSN 1064-3745 ISSN 1940-6029 (electronic)
Methods in Molecular Biology
ISBN 978-1-4939-7864-9 ISBN 978-1-4939-7865-6 (eBook)
https://doi.org/10.1007/978-1-4939-7865-6

Library of Congress Control Number: 2018940666

Printed on acid-free paper

This Humana Press imprint is published by the registered company Springer Science+Business Media, LLC part of Springer Nature.
The registered company address is: 233 Spring Street, New York, NY 10013, U.S.A.

Preface

This special edition is aimed at molecular scientist and laboratory supervisors working with multiple myeloma (MM) samples and those investigators who would like to embark on studies in this field. MM is a complex disease that in most cases cannot be cured. It not only involves genomic and phenotypic alterations of plasma cells but also implicates the entire bone marrow microenvironment. The complex nature of the pathogenesis of this disease demands that great care is taken during the acquisition, isolation, and archiving of samples and the choice of molecular methods for the analysis of target cell populations, including the selection of adequate quality controls. This edition of Molecular Methods will provide an end-to-end guide from sample acquisition to the performance of molecular tests and will highlight pitfalls in quality control and interpretation of the results.

Novel agents have dramatically increased response rates in MM patients. As a result, the quality of response is increasingly being assessed by molecular tests. In Chapters 1 and 2 sophisticated and highly sensitive PCR- and next-generation-flow-based methods for detection of minimal residual disease and circulating tumor cells are described. Chapter 3 outlines a simple flow cytometry approach, which allows to determine the DNA content of MM cells and to distinguish them from normal polyclonal plasma cells. Only recently, mass cytometry has emerged as a new state-of-the-art technology application that overcomes the challenges of flow cytometry by using heavy metal ion tags. Chapter 4 describes the application of Cytometry by Time-of-Flights (CyTOF) to deeply phenotype MM samples in a clinical setting.

Advances in molecular biology methods, especially the introduction of next-generation sequencing (NGS) based approaches, have significantly improved our understanding of MM. However, the legacy method fluorescence in-situ hybridization (FISH) continues to play an important role in the detection of genomic aberrations in MM cells. In Chapter 5 the creation of custom-made DNA probes for FISH and the hybridization on various cell and tissue types are described. The application of the NGS based methods whole exome sequencing, and RNA-sequencing on low-input clinical samples is described in Chapters 6 and 7. A clinically oriented targeted NGS approach for the molecular characterization of MM is presented in Chapter 8. Recent studies have shown that MM patients frequently present with genomic variation between individual cancer foci, also termed spatial heterogeneity. As a result, genomic profiles for tumor cells from the iliac crest are not necessarily representative. In Chapter 9, a method is described which may overcome this issue by analyzing circulating cell-free tumor DNA.

The increasing applicability and sensitivity of NGS exacerbate a main issue in molecular biology, namely cross-sample contamination. A droplet digital PCR approach and a simple bioinformatics solution for the detection of contamination in patient's samples and derived sequencing data are described in Chapter 10.

Large amounts of gene expression profiling (GEP) data are publicly available. Despite the increasing significance and the advantages of RNA sequencing, GEP could still help to improve our understanding of biological processes in MM. Chapter 11 describes easy-to-use and open-access bioinformatic tools to extract and visualize important information from these profiles.

Expression profiles of MM cells are not only impacted by structural aberrations and mutations but also by epigenetic mechanisms. In Chapters 12 and 13 a method for a genome-wide investigation of the methylation and hydroxymethylation status of cytosines, and a comprehensive yet economic approach of mapping whole genome DNA methylation, optimized for MM clinical samples, are described.

Nanoparticles are the topic of the last two chapters. Chapter 14 describes a method for preparing lipid nanoparticles loaded with siRNA, mRNA, or plasmids and provides guidelines for their application to cultured cells in a well-plate format. Chapter 15 outlines a microfluidic approach for creating nanoparticles, which allows for an efficient encapsulation of both hydrophobic and hydrophilic drugs.

We are grateful to our authors for sharing their protocols. We also would like to thank the series editor, John M. Walker, Professor Emeritus in the School of Life Sciences at the University of Hertfordshire, and the editors Anna Rakovsky and David C. Casey at Springer for their support.

Spring House, PA, USA *Christoph Heuck*
Little Rock, AR, USA *Niels Weinhold*

Contents

Preface .... *v*
Contributors .... *ix*

1 ELDA qASO-PCR for High Sensitivity Detection of Tumor Cells in Bone Marrow and Peripheral Blood 1
Stefanie Huhn

2 Retracted Chapter: EuroFlow-Based Next-Generation Flow Cytometry for Detection of Circulating Tumor Cells and Minimal Residual Disease in Multiple Myeloma 15
Leire Burgos and Bruno Paiva

3 Cytoplasmic Immunoglobulin Vs. DNA Analysis by Flow Cytometry 35
Daisy Alapat

4 Deep Profiling of the Immune System of Multiple Myeloma Patients Using Cytometry by Time-of-Flight (CyTOF) 47
Tina Smets, Frederik Stevenaert, HC Adams 3rd, and Greet Vanhoof

5 Fluorescence In Situ Hybridization (FISH) in Multiple Myeloma 55
Erming Tian

6 Whole Exome Sequencing in Multiple Myeloma to Identify Somatic Single Nucleotide Variants and Key Translocations Involving Immunoglobulin Loci and MYC 71
Brian A. Walker

7 RNA-Sequencing from Low-Input Material in Multiple Myeloma for Application in Clinical Routine 97
Anja Seckinger, Tomi Bähr-Ivacevic, Vladimir Benes, and Dirk Hose

8 Protocol for M^{3}P: A Comprehensive and Clinical Oriented Targeted Sequencing Panel for Routine Molecular Analysis in Multiple Myeloma 117
Santiago Barrio, Matteo DáVia, Laura Bruins, Thorsten Stühmer, Torsten Steinbrunn, Max Bittrich, Hermann Einsele, Alexander Keith Stewart, Esteban Braggio, and Klaus Martin Kortüm

9 Analysis of Circulating Tumor DNA 129
Sridurga Mithraprabhu and Andrew Spencer

10 Detection of Cross-Sample Contamination in Multiple Myeloma Samples and Sequencing Data 147
Owen W. Stephens, Tobias Meißner, and Niels Weinhold

11 Analysis of Global Gene Expression Profiles 157
Alboukadel Kassambara and Jerome Moreaux

12 Genome Wide Mapping of Methylated and Hydroxyl-Methylated Cytosines Using a Modified HpaII Tiny Fragment Enrichment by Ligation Mediated PCR Tagged Sequencing Protocol. 167
Sanchari Battachariyya, Ruslana Tytarenko, Christoph Heuck, John Greally, and Amit Verma

13 A Rapid and Robust Protocol for Reduced Representation Bisulfite Sequencing in Multiple Myeloma 179
Samrat Roy Choudhury and Brian A. Walker

14 Microfluidic Production and Application of Lipid Nanoparticles for Nucleic Acid Transfection 193
Anitha Thomas, Shyam M. Garg, Rebecca A. G. De Souza, Eric Ouellet, Grace Tharmarajah, Dave Reichert, Mina Ordobadi, Shell Ip, and Euan C. Ramsay

15 Microfluidic Assembly of Liposomes with Tunable Size and Coloading Capabilities. 205
Jessica R. Hoffman, Ennio Tasciotti, and Roberto Molinaro

Retraction Note to: EuroFlow-Based Next-Generation Flow Cytometry for Detection of Circulating Tumor Cells and Minimal Residual Disease E1

Correction to: Multiple Myeloma E3

Index. 215

Contributors

HC Adams 3RD · *Janssen Research and Development, LLC, Spring House, PA, USA*

Daisy Alapat · *Department of Pathology, University of Arkansas for Medical Sciences, Little Rock, AR, USA*

Tomi Bähr-Ivacevic · *Labor für Myelomforschung, Medizinische Klinik V, Universitätsklinikum Heidelberg, Heidelberg, Germany*

Santiago Barrio · *Department of Internal Medicine II, University Hospital Würzburg, Würzburg, Germany*

Sanchari Battachariyya · *Albert Einstein College of Medicine, Bronx, NY, USA*

Vladimir Benes · *Genomics Core Facility, European Molecular Biology Laboratory, Heidelberg, Germany*

Max Bittrich · *Department of Internal Medicine II, University Hospital Würzburg, Würzburg, Germany*

Esteban Braggio · *Department of Hematology and Oncology, Mayo Clinic, Scottsdale, AZ, USA*

Laura Bruins · *Department of Hematology and Oncology, Mayo Clinic, Scottsdale, AZ, USA*

Leire Burgos · *Universidad De Navarra, Pamplona, Spain*

Samrat Roy Choudhury · *Department of Internal Medicine, Myeloma Institute, University of Arkansas for Medical Sciences, Little Rock, AR, USA*

Matteo DáVia · *Department of Internal Medicine II, University Hospital Würzburg, Würzburg, Germany*

Rebecca A. G. De Sousa · *Precision NanoSystems, Vancouver, BC, Canada*

Hermann Einsele · *Department of Internal Medicine II, University Hospital Würzburg, Würzburg, Germany*

Shyam M. Garg · *Precision NanoSystems, Vancouver, BC, Canada*

John Greally · *Albert Einstein College of Medicine, Bronx, NY, USA*

Christoph Heuck · *Janssen R&D, Spring House, PA, USA*

Jessica R. Hoffman · *University of North Carolina, Chapel Hill, NC, USA; Center for Biomimetic Medicine, Houston Methodist Research Institute, Houston, TX, USA*

Dirk Hose · *Labor für Myelomforschung, Medizinische Klinik V, Universitätsklinikum Heidelberg, Heidelberg, Germany*

Stefanie Huhn · *Department of Internal Medicine V, University of Heidelberg, Heidelberg, Germany*

Shell Ip · *Precision NanoSystems, Vancouver, BC, Canada*

Alboukadel Kassambara · *Department of Biological Hematology, CHU Montpellier, Montpellier, France; Institute of Human Genetics, UMR 9002, CNRS and University of Montpellier, Montpellier, France*

Klaus Martin Kortüm · *Department of Internal Medicine II, University Hospital Würzburg, Würzburg, Germany*

Tobias Meißner · *Department of Molecular and Experimental Medicine, Avera Cancer Institute, Sioux Falls, SD, USA*

Sridurga Mithraprabhu · *Myeloma Research Group, Australia Centre for Blood Diseases, Alfred Hospital—Monash University, Melbourne, VIC, Australia; Malignant Haematology and Stem Cell Transplantation, Alfred Hospital, Melbourne, VIC, Australia*

Roberto Molinaro · *Center for Biomimetic Medicine, Houston Methodist Research Institute, Houston, TX, USA; Department of Medicine, Cardiovascular Medicine, Harvard Medical School Brigham and Women's Hospital, Boston, MA, USA*

Jerome Moreaux · *Department of Biological Hematology, CHU Montpellier, Montpellier, France; Institute of Human Genetics, UMR 9002, CNRS and University of Montpellier, Montpellier, France; UFR de Medicine, University of Montpellier, Montpellier, France; Department of Biological Hematology, Laboratory for Monitoring Innovative Therapies, Hopital Saint-Eloi—CHRU de Montpellier, Montpellier, France*

Mina Ordobadi · *Precision NanoSystems, Vancouver, BC, Canada*

Eric Ouellet · *Precision NanoSystems, Vancouver, BC, Canada*

Bruno Paiva · *Universidad De Navarra, Pamplona, Spain*

Euan C. Ramsay · *Precision NanoSystems, Vancouver, BC, Canada*

Dave Reichert · *Precision NanoSystems, Vancouver, BC, Canada*

Anja Seckinger · *Labor für Myelomforschung, Medizinische Klinik V, Universitätsklinikum Heidelberg, Heidelberg, Germany*

Tina Smets · *Janssen Research and Development, Beerse, Belgium*

Andrew Spencer · *Myeloma Research Group, Australian Centre for Blood Diseases, Alfred Hospital-Monash University, Melbourne, VIC, Australia; Malignant Haematology and Stem Cell Transplantation, Alfred Hospital, Melbourne, VIC, Australia; Department of Clinical Haematology, Monash University, Melbourne, VIC, Australia*

Torsten Steinbrunn · *Department of Internal Medicine II, University Hospital Würzburg, Würzburg, Germany*

Owen W. Stephens · *The Myeloma Institute, University of Arkansas for Medical Sciences, Little Rock, AR, USA*

Frederick Stevenaert · *Janssen Research and Development, Beerse, Belgium*

Alexander Keith Stewart · *Department of Hematology and Oncology, Mayo Clinic, Scottsdale, AZ, USA; Center for Individualized Medicine, Mayo Clinic, Rochester, MN, USA*

Thorsten Stühmer · *Department of Internal Medicine II, University Hospital Würzburg, Würzburg, Germany*

Ennio Tasciotti · *Center for Biomimetic Medicine, Houston Methodist Research Institute, Houston, TX, USA; Houston Methodist Orthopedics and Sports Medicine, Institute for Academic Medicine, Houston Methodist Research Institute, Houston, TX, USA*

Grace Tharmarajah · *Precision NanoSystems, Vancouver, BC, Canada*

Anitha Thomas · *Precision NanoSystems, Vancouver, BC, Canada*

Erming Tian · *Myeloma Institute, University of Arkansas for Medical Sciences, Little Rock, AR, USA*

Ruslana Tytarenko · *University of Arkansas for Medical Sciences, Little Rock, AR, USA*

Greet Vanhoof · *Janssen Research and Development, Beerse, Belgium*

Amit Verma · *Albert Einstein College of Medicine, Bronx, NY, USA*

Brian A. Walker · *Department of Internal Medicine, Myeloma Institute, University of Arkansas for Medical Sciences, Little Rock, AR, USA*

Niels Weinhold · *The Myeloma Institute, University of Arkansas for Medical Sciences, Little Rock, AR, USA*

Chapter 1

ELDA qASO-PCR for High Sensitivity Detection of Tumor Cells in Bone Marrow and Peripheral Blood

Stefanie Huhn

Abstract

A quantitative allele-specific polymerase chain reaction in combination with an extreme limiting dilution approach (ELDA qASO-PCR) enables the detection of tumor cells in patients with multiple myeloma (MM) in bone marrow (BM) samples and in peripheral blood (PB) with a sensitivity of $<10^{-6}$. The two-step procedure of patient-specific tumor cell identification via the immunoglobulin heavy chain (IgH) and kappa/lambda light chain (k/λ LC) locus, followed by tumor cells quantification by ELDA qASO-PCR allows for the application of this method to the majority of MM patients, including those with Bence Jones proteinuria.

Key words qASO-PCR, Minimal residual diseases, Multiple myeloma

1 Introduction

Multiple myeloma (MM) is characterized by the accumulation of malignant plasma cells (PC) in the bone marrow (BM). The detection and quantification of these PC plays an important role, not only for diagnosis of MM but also for the evaluation of response to therapy [1]. Small numbers of residual tumor cells (minimal residual disease, MRD) that have not been eliminated by therapy are the cause of relapse of the disease even in patients who achieve clinical complete response (CR) [1]. Accordingly, the presence of MRD in these patients is associated with a worse progression free and overall survival [2–7]. Highly sensitive methods for detection of MRD, such as multicolor flow cytometry (MFC), allele-specific oligonucleotide PCR (ASO-PCR) and next generation sequencing (NGS) based assays, enable detection of residual tumor cells.

The quantitative allele-specific polymerase chain reaction in combination with an extreme limiting dilution approach (ELDA qASO-PCR) is a molecular method for MRD-detection that reaches very high sensitivities and is able to detect one tumor cell among one million normal mononuclear cells. It can be applied to

Christoph Heuck and Niels Weinhold (eds.), *Multiple Myeloma: Methods and Protocols*, Methods in Molecular Biology, vol. 1792, https://doi.org/10.1007/978-1-4939-7865-6_1,

BM aspirates for MRD-diagnosis and to PB for the detection and quantification of circulating tumor cells (CTCs).

The two-step procedure of patient-specific tumor cell identification via the immunoglobulin heavy chain (IgH) and kappa/lambda light chain (k/λ LC) locus, followed by tumor cell quantification by ELDA qASO-PCR allows for the application of this method to the majority of MM patients, including those with Bence Jones proteinuria.

2 Material

2.1 Identification of Tumor-Specific Immunoglobulin Rearrangement

1. CD138-enriched PCs from BM aspirates collected at the time of diagnosis [8].
2. DNA/RNA Extraction kit.
3. cDNA Synthesis kit.
4. Agarose gel (*see* **Note 1**).
5. 1× TAE Buffer (100 mL 50× TAE + 4900 mL molecular grade H_2O).
6. Molecular grade H_2O.
7. Gel Stain (adjusted 1 μL gel stain to 1 g of agarose).
8. DNA ladder (50 bp).
9. 6× DNA loading dye.
10. Compact Multi-Wide Horizontal Gel Electrophoresis Apparatus.
11. PCR reaction reagents (*see* Table 1).
12. Consensus Primer (sequence *see* Table 2).
13. High pure PCR product purification kit.
14. Sequencing Primer (*see* Primer sequences).
15. Standard in-house or core facility reagents for Sanger sequencing.

2.2 Design of the Patient-Specific PCR Reaction

1. cDNA from CD138-enriched PCs.
2. PCR reaction reagents (*see* Table 3).
3. Patient-specific primers.

2.3 Tumor Cell Quantification

1. Unsorted BM aspirate or PB sample in EDTA.
2. 15 mL Ficoll-Hypaque solution per sample.
3. 1× PBS + EDTA: 900 mL H_2O + 100 mL 10× phosphate-buffered saline (PBS) + 4 mL EDTA (0.5 mM).
4. DNA extraction kit.
5. Agarose gel (*see* **Note 1**).

Table 1
Consensus PCR reaction mix

Reagents per sample	μL				
10× buffer[a]	2.5				
MgCl[a] 25 mM	2	**PCR conditions**			
dNTPs (20 mM each)	1	**IgH**		**k/λ LC**	
Primer forward 20 mM	0.5	95 °C × 5 min		95 °C × 5 min	
Primer reverse 20 mM	0.5	95 °C × 30 s	35×	94 °C × 30 s	40×
H_2O	17.25	63 °C × 30 s		60 °C × 45 s	
Taq polymerases[b]	0.25	72 °C × 30 s		72 °C × 45 s	
cDNA from CD138-enriched PCs	1	72 °C × 5 min		72 °C × 10 min	
Final volume	25				

[a]As recommended for the used Taq Polymerases
[b]We highly recommend AmpliTaq Gold by Invitrogen which showed best results of all tested Taq Polymerases

Table 2
Consensus primer sequences

Location	Orientation	Name	Primer sequence
IgH	Forward	FR1C	GGTGCAGCTGSWGSAGTCDGG
	Reverse	LJH-CL	CTCGCTCGCCCATGAGGAGACGGTGACC
Kappa	Forward	VKKL1a	GGA GAC AGA GTC ACC ATC ACT TG
		VKKL2a	CTC CAT CTC CTG CAG GTC TAG
		VKKL3a	CTG CAG GGC CAG TCA GAG
		VKKL5a	CTT TGT CTC CTG GAG TCG CTG
	Reverse	JKKL4123	GTT TGA TCT CCA CCT TGG TCC C
		JKKL5	TCG AGT CCC TTG GCC GAA GGT G
Lambda	Forward	VLKL12a	GGT CCT GGG CTC AGT CTG
		VLKL3c	TGG TAC CAG CAG AAG CCA GG
		VLKL4a	CCA GCC TGT GCT GAC TCA
		VLKL7a	CAG ACT GTG GTG ACT CAG GAG
	Reverse	JLHD123	CTA GGA CGG TGA GCT TGG TCC C
		JLKL4	GAC TCA TCT AAA ATG ATC AGC TGG G
		JLKL5	AGA CTC ATC TAG GAC GGT CAG

Table 3
PCR reaction mix for primer temperature and specificity test and primer sensitivity test

Temperature and specificity test		Sensitivity test			
Reagents per sample	**µL**	**Reagents per sample**	**µL**		
10× buffer[a]	5	10× buffer[a]	5		
MgCl[a] 25 mM	4	MgCl[a] 25 mM	4		
dNTPs 20 mM each	2	dNTPs 20 mM each	2		
Primer FW 20 mM	2	Primer FW 20 mM	2	**PCR conditions**	
Primer RW 20 mM	2	Primer RW 20 mM	2	95 °C × 5 min	
High pure H_2O	23.5	High pure H_2O	23.5	95 °C × 30 s	40×
Taq[b]	0.5	Taq[b]	0.5	Annealing[c] × 30 s	
Buffy coat DNA 100 ng/µL or H_2O	10	Buffy coat DNA 100 ng/µL or H_2O	10	72 °C × 30 s	
Product of consensus PCR 10^5 copies	1	Product of consensus PCR Dilution series	1	72 °C 5 min	
Final volume	50	Final volume	50		

[a]As recommended for the used Taq polymerases; FW forward primer mix; RW reverse primer mix
[b]We recommend AmpliTaq Gold by Invitrogen which showed best results of all tested Taq polymerases
[c]Annealing temperature according to test

6. 1× TAE Buffer (100 mL 50× TAE + 4900 mL molecular grade H_2O).
7. Molecular grade H_2O.
8. Gel Stain (volume adjusted 1 µL gel stain to 1 g of agarose).
9. DNA ladder (50 bp).
10. 6× DNA loading dye.
11. Compact Multi-Wide horizontal gel electrophoresis apparatus.
12. A minimum of 6 µg genomic DNA of patient sample (full PB or BM) for diagnostics.
13. PCR reaction reagents (*see* Table 4).
14. Patient-specific primers.
15. Sequence alignment software (e.g., MEGA).
16. R. packages NADA and ggplot2.
17. Browser tools: "VBASE2" (http://www.vbase2.org/) and "ELDA: Extreme Limiting Dilution Analysis" (http://bioinf.wehi.edu.au/software/elda/).

Table 4
PCR reaction mix for quantification of tumor cells in patient samples

Quantification				
Reagents per sample	**µL**			
10× buffer[a]	5			
MgCl[a] 25 mM	4			
dNTPs 20 mM each	2	**PCR conditions**		
Primer FW 20 mM	2	95 °C × 5 min		
Primer RW 20 mM	2	95 °C × 30 s	Standard 40× + 10	Nested 25×
High pure H_2O	24.5	Annealing[b] × 30 s		
Taq[c]	0.5	72 °C × 30 s		
DNA of patient sample Dilution series	10	72 °C 5 min		
Final volume	50			

[a]As recommended for the used Taq polymerases; FW forward primer mix; RW reverse primer mix
[b]Annealing temperature according to temperature test
[c]We recommend AmpliTaq Gold by Invitrogen which showed best results of all tested Taq polymerases

3 Methods

3.1 Identification of Tumor-Specific Immunoglobulin Rearrangement

1. Isolate DNA & RNA from CD138-enriched PCs from BM aspirates [8] collected at time of diagnosis using a DNA/RNA extraction kit according to the manufacturer's recommendations.
2. Synthesize cDNA from 10 to 50 ng of RNA using a cDNA synthesis kit according to the manufacturer's recommendations.
3. Use cDNA as template for the consensus PCR reaction (Reagents and protocol Table 1).
4. We suggest a two-step approach by first carrying out the consensus PCR for the IgH locus and only perform the consensus PCR of the k/λ LC locus, if the consensus PCR for the IgH locus fails to amplify a monoclonal sequence (*see* **Note 2**).
5. Check amplification success on a 2% agarose gel.
6. Clean up PCR product with a high pure PCR product purification kit.
7. Measure concentration of the cleanup PCR product by optical density (OD) measurement.
8. Sequence the PCR product. Sanger sequencing of the PCR product of the consensus PCR can be performed in-house or

be outsourced to a sequencing core facility. Requirements for sequencing primers and PCR products have to be prepared according to the in-house or core facility sequencing protocols (*see* **Note 3**).

3.2 Design of the Patient-Specific PCR Reaction

1. Align FASTA files from forward and reverse Sanger sequencing using a sequencing alignment program such as MEGA ([9] free ware) and check for inconsistencies.
2. Import the final sequence into the VBASE2 browser, which is an integrative database of germ-line variable genes from the immunoglobulin loci of human and mouse based on EMBL-Bank [10].
3. Retrieve nucleotide alignment of patient sequence and banked IgH or k/λ LC. Design primer pairs binding at complementary determining region (CDR) 1 or 2 (forward primer) and CDR3 (reverse primer), where the patient nucleotide sequence varies from as many aligned IgH or k/λ LC sequences as possible. The 3′ end of each primer should hit at least one sequence variation, preferably two or more. Adjust length of the primer towards the 5′ end in order to reach matching annealing temperatures for all primer pairs.
4. We recommend designing—whenever possible—at least two primer pairs to allow for a nested PCR (Fig. 1) and favor higher annealing temperatures of >60 °C for higher specificity of the primer.
5. Perform PCR reaction using the cleanup PCR product of the initial consensus PCR with 10^5 copies/μL as positive control and Buffy coat DNA from normal donors as negative control (Reagents and protocol Table 3; consensus PCR product dilutions Table 5).
6. For each primer pair carry out four reactions: (1) Negative control, (2) 1 μg Buffy coat DNA, (3) 10^5 copies of consensus PCR-product, and (4) 10^5 copies of consensus PCR-product plus 1 μg Buffy coat (Fig. 2).
7. We suggest carrying out the primer test at 2–3 different annealing temperatures starting with the estimated temperature of the primer synthesis and adding 2 °C (*see* **Note 4**).
8. Check PCR products on agarose gel for optimal annealing temperature and specificity (Fig. 2, *see* **Note 1**).
9. A primer pair is considered specific if a single distinct band with the correct length is visible for the positive control and no amplification is visible using Buffy Coat DNA as template.
10. Select a specific primer pair for the following sensitivity test, keeping in mind an optional nested PCR.
11. Test the sensitivity of the preferred primer pair by stepwise diluting the cleanup PCR product of the initial consensus

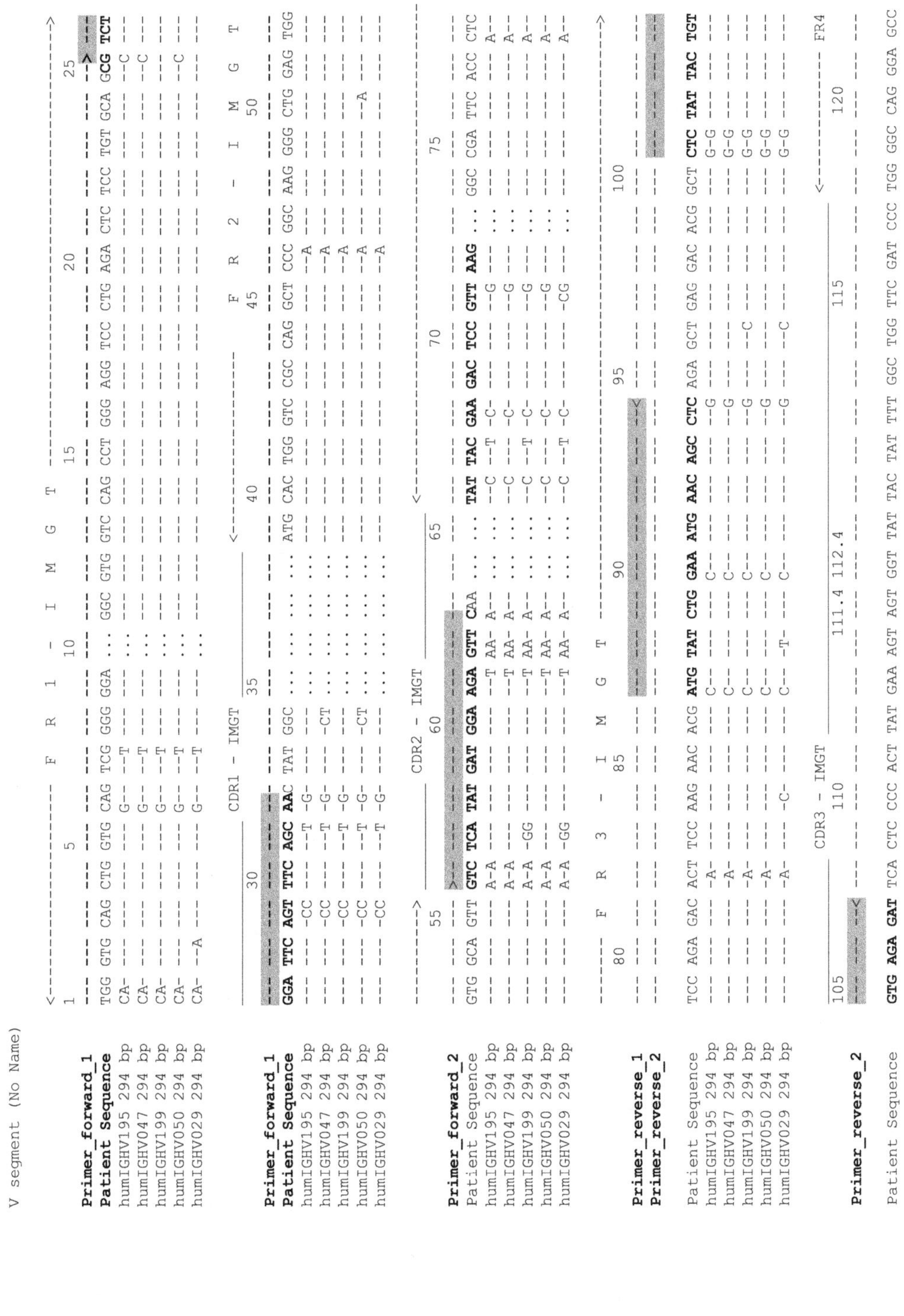

Fig. 1 Primer design example for an IgH sequence

Table 5
Preparation of consensus PCR product dilutions for primer temperature and specificity test and primer sensitivity test and for positive controls

Length of fragment	bp	A
Molecular weight/bp	g/mol	660
Molecular weight/fragment		$B = A \div 660$
ag/mol fragment	ag/mol	$C = B \times 10^{18}$
Weight/fragment	ng/µl	D
Weight/molecule	ag/molecule	$E = C \times (6.023 \times 10^{18})$
Dilution factor for 1×10^9 molecules/µL		$F = E \times D$
Clean up PCR-product	µL	1
TE-buffer	µL	$G = F - 1$
Log dilution steps	*Template copies*	
1:10	1×10^8	
1:10	1×10^7	
1:10	1×10^6	
1:10	1×10^5	
1:10	1×10^3	
1:10	1000	
1:10	100	
1:10	10	
1:10	1	

PCR from 10^5 copies to one template molecule per reaction mix (consensus PCR product dilutions Table 5; Fig. 2).

12. Carry out this dilution series twice: (1) in H_2O and (2) with 1 µg Buffy Coat DNA added to each reaction and perform PCR reaction according to the protocol shown in Table 3.
13. Check PCR products on an agarose gel after 40 PCR cycles (Fig. 2, *see* **Note 1**).
14. A PCR assay is considered sensitive if (1) a distinct band of amplification with the correct length is visible on the gel down to the dilution of one template molecule per reaction, and (2) no unspecific amplification product is visible on the gel (Fig. 2).
15. The sensitivity may be increased by ten additional cycles or a nested PCR design. For a nested PCR, dilute PCR product of the previous reaction 1:50 and use 1 µL of the dilution as template for a PCR with a second set of primers. Check PCR products on an agarose gel (*see* **Note 1**).

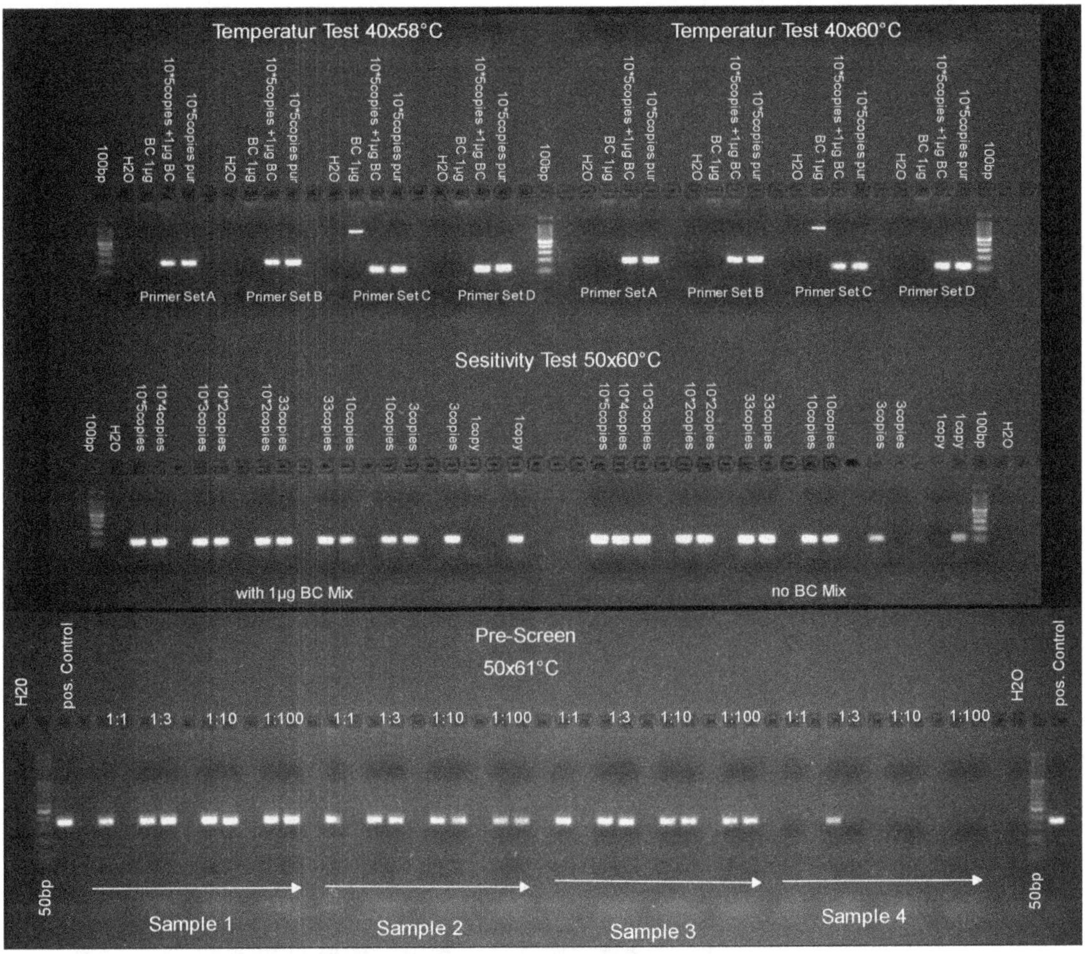

Fig. 2 Agarose gel picture of primer temperature and specificity test, primer sensitivity test and prescreen results of a quantification of tumor cells in patient samples

3.3 Tumor Cell Quantification

1. Obtain mononuclear cells from patient samples (whole blood or bone marrow) by Ficoll-Hypaque density centrifugation.
2. Use 15 mL Ficoll solution and 35 mL patient sample suspended in PBS + EDTA buffer (adapted to volume of sample material) for density centrifugation (30 min at 1578 × *g*, without break).
3. Remove interphase and wash in 40 mL 1× PBS + EDTA (10 min at 652 × *g*, with break).
4. Discard liquid phase and suspend cell pellet in 1.6 mL 1× PBS + EDTA and transfer to storage tube. Spin for 30 s at 17000 × *g* and discard liquid phase.
5. From the cell pellet, genomic DNA is isolated using the QIAamp DNA Blood Kit (Qiagen) according to the manufacturer's recommendations and quantified by optical density (OD) measurement.

6. After Ficoll-Hypaque density centrifugation as well as after genomic DNA isolation samples should be stored at −20 °C (*see* **Note 5**).
7. Check integrity and quality of the DNA by (1) OD measurement for sample purity (260:280 and 260:230 ratios), (2) a low density agarose gel (1%), and (3) a reference PCR reaction before quantification as described [11].
8. Perform PCR reactions for quantification of residual tumor cells: start with a prescreen of the sample in a short duplicate dilution series ideally 1 μg (~165,000 cells), 333 ng and 100 ng templates DNA per 50 μL PCR reaction (reagents and protocol in Table 4; Fig. 2). In each PCR carry two H_2O negative controls and the cleanup PCR product of the initial consensus PCR (10^5 copies/μL) as positive control (consensus PCR product dilutions shown in Table 5).
9. Check PCR products on an agarose gel (*see* **Note 1**).
10. Samples that are negative in the prescreen should be tested using >1.000.000 cells (~7 μg DNA) in additional short dilution series to assure the high sensitivity of $\leq 10^{-6}$ (Examples in Table 6).
11. For samples that show amplification in the prescreen, the screening should be continued. Dilute the series in log steps (1:10, 1:100, 1:1000, etc.) until reaching a negative dilution step. At this point repeat the previous reaction for confirmation with a minimum number of 10 duplicates for the negative (0/10) dilution step (Examples in Table 6).
12. Carry out follow up reactions always starting from the last dilution step that was positive in all duplicates of the previous reaction with five duplicates for each additional dilution step (Examples in Table 6, *see* **Note 6**).
13. Include 1:3 dilution steps as soon as the dilution shows incomplete amplifications in duplications (Examples in Table 6).
14. To determine the proportion of tumor cells per sample use the "ELDA: Extreme Limiting Dilution Analysis" (http://bioinf.wehi.edu.au/software/elda/) software [12] and the quantification results as input.
15. For group comparisons of tumor cell loads we recommend the R package NADA [13] for left-censored data. Using this approach MRD-negative results are included as censored data, using the number of tested cells as individual censoring value for each sample. Thus, strict cut-offs can be avoided, if the amount of sample material for MRD testing varies significantly between patients An example is shown in Fig. 3.
16. Correlations with clinical factors can be estimated using Kendall rank correlation coefficient with Akritas-Theil-Sen nonparametric line and the Turnbull estimate of intercept (NADA function: cenken).

Table 6
Examples of a quantification of tumor cells in patient samples

Example 1	**1:1**	**1:3**	**1:10**	**1:30**	**1:100**	**1:300**	**1:1.000**	**1:3.000**			
ng DNA per reaction	1000 ng	333 ng	100 ng	33 ng	10 ng	3.3 ng	1 ng	0.3 ng			
N cells per reaction	165,000	55,000	16,500	5500	1650	550	165	55			
Prescreen	2/2	2/2	2/2								
PCR2			2/2		5/5		2/5				
PCR3					2/2	3/5	2/5	0/5			
PCR4					2/2	3/5	2/5	0/10			
Σ	2/2	2/2	4/4		7/7	6/10	6/15	0/15			
Example 2	**1:1**	**1:3**	**1:10**	**1:30**	**1:100**	**1:300**	**1:1.000**	**1:3.000**	**1:10.000**	**1:30.000**	**1:100.000**
ng DNA per reaction	1000 ng	333 ng	100 ng	33 ng	10 ng	3.3 ng	1 ng	0.3 ng	0.1 ng	0.03 ng	0.01
N cells per reaction	165,000	55,000	16,500	5500	1650	550	165	55	17	5.5	1.7
Prescreen	2/2	2/2	2/2								
PCR2			2/2		5/5		5/5				
PCR3							2/2		5/5	1/5	0/5
PCR4									5/5	1/5	0/10
Σ	1/1	2/2	4/4		5/5		6/15		10/10	2/10	0/15
Example 3	**1:1**	**1:3**	**1:10**								
ng DNA per reaction	1000 ng	333 ng	100 ng								
N cells per reaction	165,000	55,000	16,500								
Prescreen	0/2	0/2	0/2								
PCR2	0/2	0/10	0/10	**Cells tested:**							
Σ	0/4	0/12	0/12	**1,518,000**							

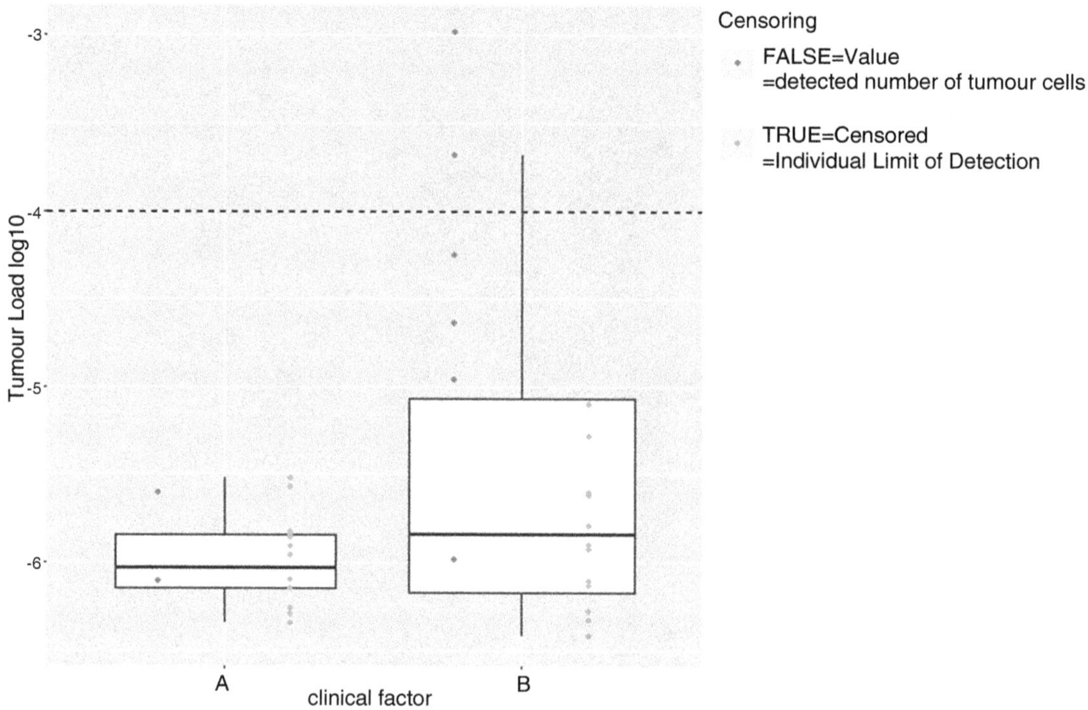

Fig. 3 Example plot for censored data: Ordinary boxplots ignoring censoring; plus scatter plot stratified for values and censored data

17. The Peto & Peto modification of the Gehan-Wilcoxon test can be used to investigate differences in the median tumor load (NADA functions cenfit & cendiff) [13].

4 Notes

1. Adjust the density of agarose gels to the fragment length for optimal separation: 200 bp 2%; 150 bp 2.5%; 100 bp 3%, and <100 bp 5%.
2. For the k/λ LC locus it is only necessary to perform sequencing for the expressed LC.
3. Sequencing should always be performed forward and reverse for each sample.
4. Higher temperatures may result in higher specificity of the primer set.
5. DNA extracts are more stable than cell pellets. Thus, we recommend to extract the DNA from cell pellets as soon as possible.
6. Dilutions below 0.007 ng (<1 cell) per reaction are not required.

Acknowledgments

We thank Manfed Küpper for his assistance in the design of the consensus primers for k/λ loci.

References

1. Kumar S, Paiva B, Anderson KC, Durie B, Landgren O, Moreau P, Munshi N, Lonial S, Blade J, Mateos MV, Dimopoulos M, Kastritis E, Boccadoro M, Orlowski R, Goldschmidt H, Spencer A, Hou J, Chng WJ, Usmani SZ, Zamagni E, Shimizu K, Jagannath S, Johnsen HE, Terpos E, Reiman A, Kyle RA, Sonneveld P, Richardson PG, McCarthy P, Ludwig H, Chen W, Cavo M, Harousseau JL, Lentzsch S, Hillengass J, Palumbo A, Orfao A, Rajkumar SV, San Miguel J, Avet-Loiseau H (2016) International Myeloma Working Group consensus criteria for response and minimal residual disease assessment in multiple myeloma. Lancet Oncol 17(8):e328–e346. https://doi.org/10.1016/S1470-2045(16)30206-6
2. Paiva B, Vidriales MB, Cervero J, Mateo G, Perez JJ, Montalban MA, Sureda A, Montejano L, Gutierrez NC, Garcia de Coca A, de Las Heras N, Mateos MV, Lopez-Berges MC, Garcia-Boyero R, Galende J, Hernandez J, Palomera L, Carrera D, Martinez R, de la Rubia J, Martin A, Blade J, Lahuerta JJ, Orfao A, San Miguel JF, Groups GPCS (2008) Multiparameter flow cytometric remission is the most relevant prognostic factor for multiple myeloma patients who undergo autologous stem cell transplantation. Blood 112(10):4017–4023. https://doi.org/10.1182/blood-2008-05-159624
3. Rawstron AC, Child JA, de Tute RM, Davies FE, Gregory WM, Bell SE, Szubert AJ, Navarro-Coy N, Drayson MT, Feyler S, Ross FM, Cook G, Jackson GH, Morgan GJ, Owen RG (2013) Minimal residual disease assessed by multiparameter flow cytometry in multiple myeloma: impact on outcome in the Medical Research Council Myeloma IX Study. J Clin Oncol 31(20):2540–2547. https://doi.org/10.1200/JCO.2012.46.2119
4. Korde N, Zingone A, Kwok ML, Manasanch EE, Bhutani M, Tageja N, Kazandjian D, Mailankody S, Costello R, Zhang Y, Burton D, Carter G, Wu P, Mulquin M, Zuchlinski D, Maric I, Calvo KR, Braylan RC, Roschewski M, Yuan C, Stetler-Stevenson M, Arthur DC, Lindenberg L, Kurdziel K, Choyke P, Steinberg SM, Landgren O (2013) Phase II clinical and correlative study of carfilzomib, lenalidomide, and dexamethasone followed by lenalidomide extended dosing (CRD-R) induces high rates of MRD negativity in newly diagnosed multiple myeloma (MM) patients. Blood 122(21)
5. Sherrod AM, Hari P, Mosse CA, Walker RC, Cornell RF (2015) Minimal residual disease testing after stem cell transplantation for multiple myeloma. Bone Marrow Transplant. https://doi.org/10.1038/bmt.2015.164
6. Avet-Loiseau H, Corre J, Lauwers-Cances V, Chretien M-L, Robillard N, Leleu X, Hulin C, Gentil C, Arnulf B, Belhadj K, Brechignac S, Garderet L, Karlin L, Marit G, Benboubker L, Orsini-Piocelle F, Royer B, Drenou B, Tiab M, Lamy T, MACRO M, Richardson PG, Anderson KC, Faham M, Facon T, Moreau P, Attal M, Munshi NC (2015) Evaluation of minimal residual disease (MRD) by next generation sequencing (NGS) is highly predictive of progression free survival in the IFM/DFCI 2009 trial. Blood 126(23):191
7. Martinez-Lopez J, Lahuerta JJ, Pepin F, Gonzalez M, Barrio S, Ayala R, Puig N, Montalban MA, Paiva B, Weng L, Jimenez C, Sopena M, Moorhead M, Cedena T, Rapado I, Mateos MV, Rosinol L, Oriol A, Blanchard MJ, Martinez R, Blade J, San Miguel J, Faham M, Garcia-Sanz R (2014) Prognostic value of deep sequencing method for minimal residual disease detection in multiple myeloma. Blood 123(20):3073–3079. https://doi.org/10.1182/blood-2014-01-550020
8. Hose D, Reme T, Meissner T, Moreaux J, Seckinger A, Lewis J, Benes V, Benner A, Hundemer M, Hielscher T, Shaughnessy JD Jr, Barlogie B, Neben K, Kramer A, Hillengass J, Bertsch U, Jauch A, De Vos J, Rossi JF, Mohler T, Blake J, Zimmermann J, Klein B, Goldschmidt H (2009) Inhibition of aurora kinases for tailored risk-adapted treatment of multiple myeloma. Blood 113(18):4331–4340. https://doi.org/10.1182/blood-2008-09-178350
9. Kumar S, Stecher G, Tamura K (2016) MEGA7: molecular evolutionary genetics analysis version 7.0 for bigger datasets. Mol Biol Evol 33(7):1870–1874. https://doi.org/10.1093/molbev/msw054

10. Retter I, Althaus HH, Munch R, Muller W (2005) VBASE2, an integrative V gene database. Nucleic Acids Res 33(Database issue):D671–D674. https://doi.org/10.1093/nar/gki088
11. Cremer FW, Ehrbrecht E, Kiel K, Benner A, Hegenbart U, Ho AD, Goldschmidt H, Moos M (2000) Evaluation of the kinetics of the bone marrow tumor load in the course of sequential high-dose therapy assessed by quantitative PCR as a predictive parameter in patients with multiple myeloma. Bone Marrow Transplant 26(8):851–858. https://doi.org/10.1038/sj.bmt.1702628
12. Hu Y, Smyth GK (2009) ELDA: extreme limiting dilution analysis for comparing depleted and enriched populations in stem cell and other assays. J Immunol Methods 347(1–2):70–78. https://doi.org/10.1016/j.jim.2009.06.008
13. Helsel DR (2005) Nondectects and data analysis; statistics for censored environmental data. John Wiley and Sons, Hoboken, NJ

Chapter 2

Retracted Chapter: EuroFlow-Based Next-Generation Flow Cytometry for Detection of Circulating Tumor Cells and Minimal Residual Disease in Multiple Myeloma

Leire Burgos and Bruno Paiva

Abstract

Here, we describe the detailed protocol for minimal residual disease (MRD) assessment as well as circulating tumor cell (CTC) detection in patients with plasma cell disorders using the next-generation flow (NGF) method developed by EuroFlow. This includes the previous setup of flow cytometers, preparation and staining of samples, cell acquisition, quality control of instruments, methods and samples, as well as data interpretation to monitor MRD and CTCs with great sensitivity. It should be noted that the NGF method fully described below can be equally applied to monitor MRD in patients with systemic light-chain amyloidosis and to detect occult bone marrow involvement in patients with solitary plasmocytoma.

Key words Flow cytometry, Minimal residual disease, Circulating tumor cells, Multiple myeloma, EuroFlow, Next-generation flow

1 Introduction

Next-generation flow (NGF) cytometry is a highly sensitive and standardized method developed by EuroFlow for detection of minimal residual disease (MRD) in multiple myeloma (MM) [1]. EuroFlow is a consortium that works for the standardization and validation of highly sensitive flow cytometric tests for diagnosis and prognostic subclassification of hematological malignancies as well as for evaluation of treatment efficacy. Based on the results of its multidisciplinary translational research, EuroFlow has developed optimized and standardized instrument setup and immunostaining protocols for the diagnosis, classification, and prognostic subclassification of hematological malignancies. More recently, EuroFlow is following the same methodological approach to develop protocols for MRD detection [1, 2]. In the most recent International

The original version of this chapter was revised. The correction to this chapter is available at https://doi.org/10.1007/978-1-4939-7865-6_16

Christoph Heuck and Niels Weinhold (eds.), *Multiple Myeloma: Methods and Protocols*, Methods in Molecular Biology, vol. 1792, https://doi.org/10.1007/978-1-4939-7865-6_2, © Springer Science+Business Media, LLC, part of Springer Nature 2018

Myeloma Working Group guidelines for response assessment, new MRD criteria were introduced and MRD assessed by NGF was included [3]. On the other hand, detection and quantification of circulating tumor cells (CTCs) in the peripheral blood (PB) of patients with monoclonal gammopathies of undetermined significance (MGUS) [4], smoldering [5], and active MM has become a biomarker to predict risk of progression [6–8].

Flow cytometry is an attractive technique for the study of biological samples containing plasma cells (PCs). The principle on which it is based is simple: the biological cells or particles to be analyzed are labeled with antibodies bound to fluorochromes, suspended in an isotonic fluid flow, pushed through, and aligned one by one at high speed (up to thousands of cells per second) ahead of light beams. From the impact of light beams on each cell (i.e., lasers of specific wavelength), information is obtained from light scattering and excitation of the fluorochromes conjugated to the antibodies. This information is collected by detectors that can measure such information, and converted it into electronic signals that are finally digitized. This allows the simultaneous measurement of several parameters in the same cell or particle, a semiquantitative analysis of antigenic expression, and detection of both surface and intracellular antigens. By studying the expression of the different antigens at single-cell level, it is possible to distinguish between phenotypically normal and aberrant PCs, even when the latter are present in very low numbers (i.e., MRD or CTCs). This is possible if samples are processed using a bulk lysis methodology that allows the analysis of a significant number of cells (approximately 5×10^6 per test) without increasing the cost of the assay. Once the sample is processed and $\geq 20 \times 10^6$ cells are concentrated, they are distributed into two FACS (test) tubes where the sample is stained with combinations of eight monoclonal antibodies per test.

To date, the best strategy for identifying PCs in hematological samples is through the simultaneous analysis of CD38 and CD138. Although CD38 is widely expressed in other hematopoietic cells, its expression in PCs is bright enough to be considered a specific marker for their identification. CD138 is also a specific marker of PCs but its expression can be weaker in CTCs or even undetectable, particularly in apoptotic PCs. The detection of clonal PCs by NGF is possible through the identification of aberrant phenotypes, namely infraexpression of CD19, CD27, CD38, CD45, or CD81, overexpression of CD56, asynchronous expression of CD117, together with clonal expression of one of the two immunoglobulin light chains. According to the NGF method, the first combination aims to identify PCs (according to their expression of CD38 and/or CD138) with aberrant phenotypes (infraexpression of CD27, CD38, CD45, CD19, and/or CD81; plus, overexpression of CD56 and/or CD117). The second combination aims to demonstrate clonality (by restriction of one of the two light chains, Kappa or Lambda) in PCs previously identified according to their aberrant phenotypes. Using the Infinicyt software, both tests can be merged into a single analysis file allowing to evaluate six of the ten monoclonal antibodies simultaneously on approximately 10×10^6 cells. Therefore, this phenotypic-molecular strategy has a limit of detection of 2×10^{-6} (0,0002%; 20 tumor plasma cells) and a limit of quantification is 4×10^{-6} (0,0002%; 40 tumor cells). The availability of two tests allows to confirm the presence of low numbers of tumor cells in both tests (i.e., reproducibility). The standard operation protocol (SOP) described in detail below is valid for bone marrow (BM) aspirates and peripheral blood (PB) samples collected in EDTA tubes, and should be processed as soon as possible after sample collection, within a recommend time-frame below 36 h. Cell concentration must be assessed before any manipulation by an automated cell counter or manual counting. In order to reach the intended proposed sensitivity ($\geq 10^{-5}$), staining of at least 10×10^6 nucleated cells for each MRD tube and the systematic acquisition of more than 5×10^6 cells are required conditions.

2 Materials

Prepare all solutions using distilled H_2O at room temperature (unless indicated otherwise) and store them at 4 °C. Keep monoclonal antibodies and fluorescence beads protected from light.

1. 10× Stock solution of bulk lysis buffer: Mix 83 g of NH_4Cl, 10 g of $KHCO_3$ and 900 mL distilled H_2O in a cylinder of 1 L until all is dissolved at room temperature. Then, add 2 mL of EDTA solution and mixed thoroughly. Adjust pH of the solution with NaOH to a pH of 7.4. Precisely adjust the volume to 1 L with distilled H_2O (*see* **Note 1**).
2. Washing solution: PBS, 0.09% of NaN_3 and 0.2% BSA filtered solution (*see* **Note 2**).
3. 10× FACS Lysing solution (BD Biosciences). Dilute in distilled H_2O.
4. Fix&Perm solution (An der Grub).
5. Fluorochrome conjugated antibodies (Table 1).
6. EuroFlow Spherotech 8-peak Rainbow beads (Spherotech).
7. Compbeads (BD Biosciences).
8. FACS CantoII flow cytometer (BD Biosciences).

3 Methods

3.1 Instrument Setup

Standardization of instrument setup was developed specifically for the FACS CantoII flow cytometer. Nonetheless, the protocol can be transferred to other instruments with a minimum number of

Table 1
Technical information of Fluorochrome conjugated antibodies

Marker	Fluorochrome	Clone	Manufacturer	Catalog number
CD19	PECy7	J3-119	Beckmann Coulter	IM3628
CD27	BV510	O323	BioLegend	302835
CD38	FITC	Multi-epitope	Cytognos	CYT-38F2
CD45	PerCPCy5.5	HI30	BioLegend	304028
CD56	PE	C5.9	Cytognos	CYT-56PE
CD81	APCC750	M38	Cytognos	CYT-81AC750
CD117	APC	104D2	BD Biosciences	333233
CD138	BV421	MI15	BD Biosciences	562935
Igκ	APC	Polyclonal	Dako	C0222
Igλ	APCC750	Polyclonal	Cytognos	CYT-LAC750

Cat catalog, *PerCP* peridinin–chlorophyll–protein, *Cy5.5* cyanin5.5, *APC* allophycocyanin, *PE* phycoerythrin, *Cy7* cyanin7, *BV510* brilliant violet 510, *FITC* fluorescein isothiocyanate, *PacB* pacific blue, *C750* C750 dye, *BV421* brilliant violet 421, *Ig* immunoglobulin

requirements including. Have excitation lasers and collection optics to detect at least the eight conjugates used in the EuroFlow panel combinations, have stable fluidics, enough sensitivity to discriminate fluorescence signals, low background, signal linearity and produce data conforming to flow cytometry standard (FCS) data format.

In case of using a FACS CantoII, the FACSDiva software refers to the default configuration as the baseline one. This can be used as the template from which custom configurations can be created. In this case, a new custom configuration must be created and saved as "EuroFlow" configuration. To create the mentioned custom configuration, *see* pages 40–47 of the BD Cytometer Setup and Tracking Application Guide for BD FACS Digital Flow Cytometers [9]. An example of such configuration can be found on the EuroFlow website [10]. As far as the instrument setup is concerned, there are three items that should be done: set up Forward Scatter (FSC) and Side Scatter (SSC) parameters, set up PMT voltages for target fluorescence channels, and perform the fluorescence compensation.

1. To set up Forward Scatter (FSC) and Side Scatter (SSC) parameters, lyse 50 μL of PB from an adult healthy donor with 2 mL of 1× FACS Lysing. After an incubation for 10 min at room temperature, centrifuge for 5 min at 540 × *g*, aspirate the supernatant and then wash with 2 mL of washing solution.

After centrifugation, aspirate the supernatant and resuspend the cell pellet in 200 μL 1× PBS.

2. In the acquisition of this sample, gate lymphocytes in a FSC versus SSC bivariate dot plot and adjust FSC to the mean target value of 55.000 (range 50.000–60.000) and SSC voltage to a mean target value of 13.000 (range 11.000–15.000). Record 10.000 events.
3. To set up PMT voltages for target fluorescence channels open the FACSDiva software and create a new experiment and a worksheet with all necessary dot plots, histograms, and statistics showing the reference peak values (MFI and CV) for each fluorescence channel (*see* Fig. 1 for an illustrating example).
4. Prepare a solution containing a single drop of EuroFlow Spherotech 8-peak Rainbow beads in 1 mL of distilled H_2O and gently vortex. Acquire them (without recording) with the flow rate set at "LOW".
5. Gate single beads (*see* Population P1 in Fig. 1) in the FSC versus SSC bivariate dot plot and gate the peak of the reference target values indicated in the lot of the EuroFlow Spherotech Rainbow beads in the FITC versus PE bivariate dot plot (*see* **Note 3** and *see* Population P2 in Fig. 1).
6. Continue the acquisition and adjust PMT voltages in all fluorescence channels to reach target MFI values according to the target values of the lot of the beads used. *See* an example in the Table 2.
7. Record about 2.000 events and check the MFI for the reference peak of the beads. Once target MFI values are reached, record the target MFI achieved and the corresponding final PMT values.
8. For fluorescence compensation prepare one test tube per reagent as specified on Table 3 and stain in each tube, 50 μL of PB from an adult healthy donor with the exception of the CD138-BV421, for which one positive and one negative drop of Compbeads must be stained instead of PB. Add a "blank/unstained" tube. For Lambda APCC750 tube, three wash steps must be performed prior staining.
9. Add washing solution to reach a final volume of 100 μL per tube and mix gently.
10. Incubate for 15 min at room temperature, protected from light.
11. Add 2 mL of 1× FACS Lysing Solution and mix gently.
12. Incubate for 10 min at room temperature, protected from light.
13. Centrifuge for 5 min at 540 × *g*.

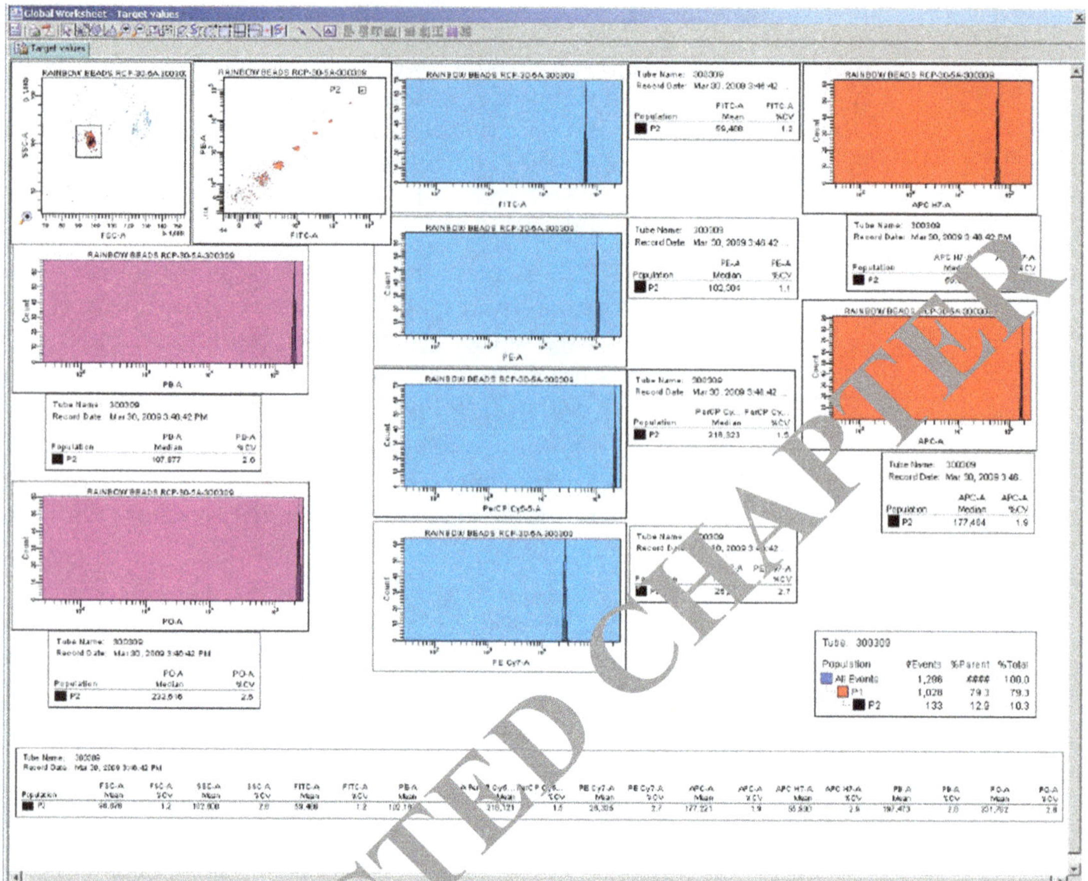

Fig. 1 Illustrating screen printout example of a worksheet with all necessary bivariate dot plots, single-parameter histograms and statistics boxes for adequate visualization of data during instrument monitoring

14. Aspirate the supernatant leaving approximately 50 μL residual volume in each tube and mix gently.
15. Add 2 mL of washing solution to each tube.
16. Centrifuge for 5 min at 540 × *g*.
17. Aspirate the supernatant leaving approximately 50 μL of residual volume in each tube and mix gently.
18. Resuspend each cell pellet with 250 μL of PBS.
19. In FACSDiva software, create a new experiment. Go to "cytometer settings" and set up the PMT voltages for FSC, SSC and all fluorescence detectors (FL1 to FL8) generated.
20. Go to "cytometer settings" and set up threshold in FSC at 10.000.
21. Go to "cytometer settings" and activate the FSC height (H) parameter.

Table 2
Example of target MFI values for the 8th peak for the different fluorochrome-matched fluorescence channels for a conventional FACSCantoII flow cytometer instrument (BD Biosciences) for 8-peak Rainbow beads lots: X02, Y02, 1016, 824430, and 45584

	Lower MFI (−15%)	Target MFI Rainbow 8-peaks (DiVa)	Upper MFI (+15%)
PacB	166,236	195,572	[illegible]
PacO	196,575	231,265	[illegible]
FITC	50,638	59,574	[illegible]
PE	86,615	101,900	117,185
PerCPCy5.5	183,654	216,064	248,474
PECy7	23,343	27,462	31,581
APC	150,263	[illegible]	203,297
APCH7	47,971	[illegible]	64,903

For other different lots check the EuroFlow website
PacB pacific blue, *PacO* pacific orange, *FITC* fluorescein isothiocyanate, *PE* phycoerythrin, *PerCP* peridinin–chlorophyll-protein, *Cy5.5* cyanin5.5, *Cy7* cyanin7, *APC* allophycocyanin

Table 3
List of fluorochrome-conjugated antibody reagents used to set up fluorescence compensation matrices

MoAb	Stain in	Notes
CD8 FITC	Peripheral blood	–
CD8 PE	Peripheral blood	–
CD45 PERCP	Peripheral blood	–
CD19 PECy7	Peripheral blood	–
CD8 APC	Peripheral blood	–
CD81 APCC750	Peripheral blood	–
LAMBDA APCC750	Peripheral blood	Perform three previous wash steps to the peripheral blood before staining
CD27 BV510	Peripheral blood	–
CD138 BV421	Compbeads	Add one drop negative and one of positive beads

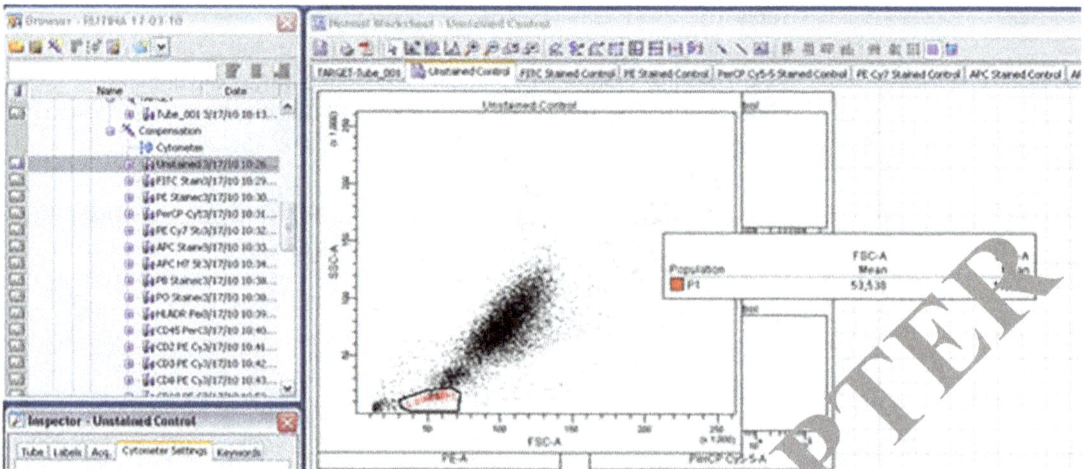

Fig. 2 Illustrating printout example of the lymphocyte gating strategy applied to the unstained compensation control tube

22. Go to "Experiment>Compensation Setup> Create compensation controls".
23. Add an additional tube for LAMBDA-APCC750 (*see* **Note 4**).
24. Acquire and record 5.000 events for the unstained control tube.
25. Gate lymphocytes in the unstained control tube as shown in Fig. 2. Then right-click with the computer's mouse over the gate region (P1) and click on "Apply to all compensation controls" option.
26. Acquire and record 5.000 events for all single stained compensation controls. The CD138-BV421 tube must be acquired at "LOW" Flow rate (*see* **Note 5**).
27. Gate lymphocytes/bead populations as illustrated in Fig. 3 in all single stained compensation control tubes (*see* **Notes 6–8**).
28. Calculate compensation: Go to Experiment>Compensation Set-up> Calculate compensation (Fig. 4).
29. Name the compensation matrix generated and then click on "Link and Save" option.

3.2 Controlling the Stability of Instruments.

Monitoring instruments performance is required to ensure the correct interpretation of results obtained and provide reproducibility of immunophenotypic studies performed at different times. This procedure must be performed daily after fluidics start-up and existing washing protocols, before acquiring samples. Instrument setup must be performed every time the cytometer configuration is changed or when the instrument does not perform under normal ranges during daily quality controls.

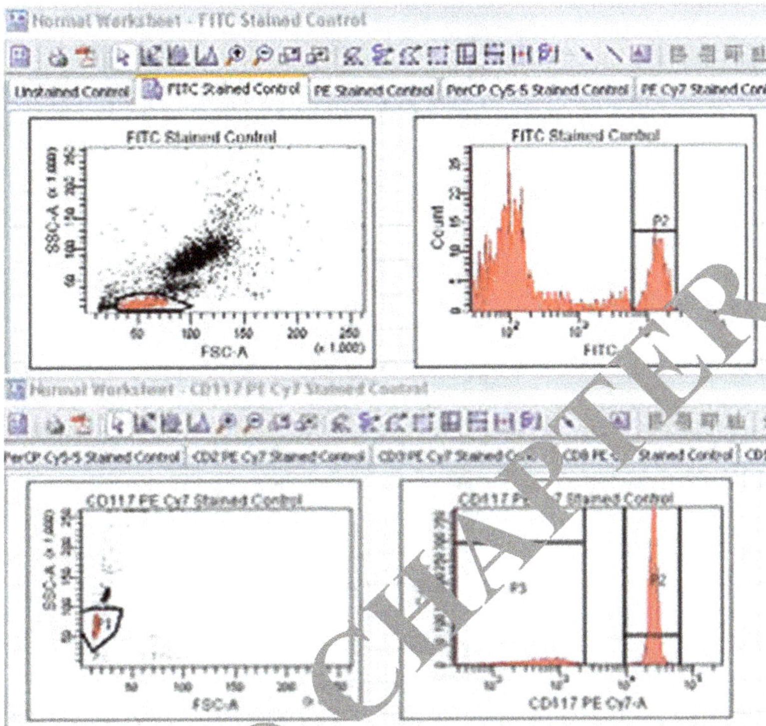

Fig. 3 Screen printout illustrating the gaiting strategy used for each single stained compensation control tube. Panel A shows an example of compensation control tubes containing PB leucocytes and panel B displays an example of compensation control tubes containing CompBeads

1. Dilute a single drop of EuroFlow Spherotech 8-peak Rainbow beads in 1 mL of distilled H_2O
2. Gently vortex and acquire them in a low flow rate.
3. Ensure that the MFI of each PMT are in the range of the target values.

3.3 Sample Preparation: Bulk Lysis

1. Transfer the sample (BM or PB) into a 50 mL Falcon tube. Do not use more than 2 mL of sample or 20×10^6 leukocytes per 50 mL of lysing solution. If more volume of sample needs to be processed (i.e., in case of starting cell concentration is low), use several 50 mL Falcon tubes.
2. Fill the tube up to reach 50 mL volume with Bulk lysis working solution.
3. Mix well and incubate for 15 min in a roller or sample-shaker device.
4. Centrifuge at $800 \times g$ for 10 min and remove the supernatant using a vacuum system without disturbing the cell pellet. No more than 300 μL of cell suspension should remain in the tube.

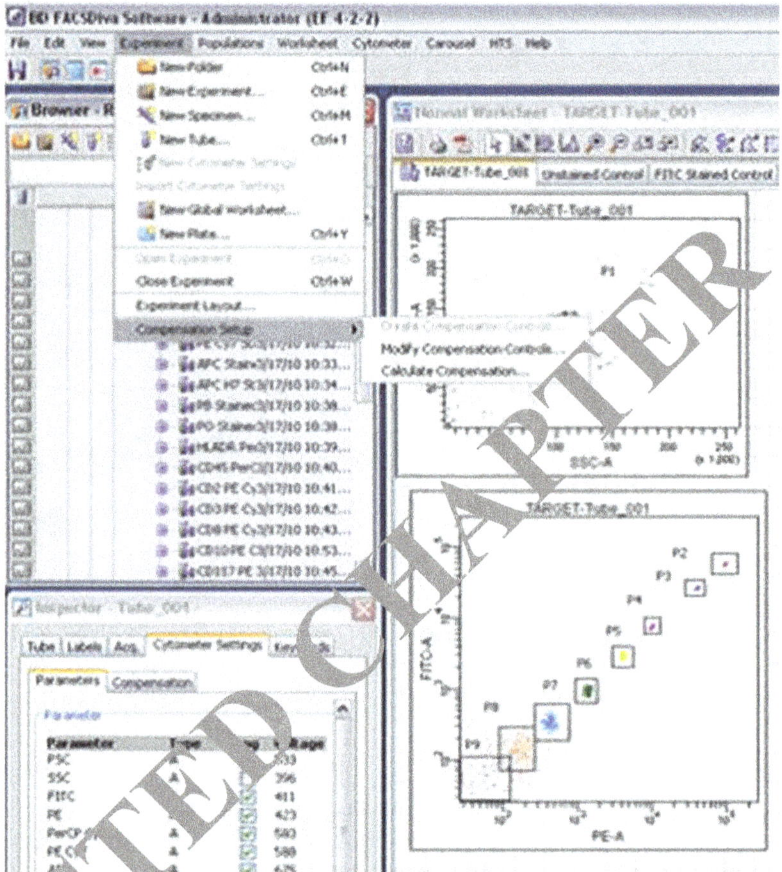

Fig. 4 Calculate compensation steps as they are visualized in the FACSDiVa software

5. Add 2 mL of washing solution and resuspend the cell pellet vigorously.
6. Complete the volume of the tube containing the cell suspension up to 50 mL of final volume with washing solution. Mix well.
7. Centrifuge at 800 × *g* for 5 min and remove the supernatant using a vacuum system, without disturbing the cell pellet.
8. Resuspend the cell pellet in 2 mL of washing solution, mix well and transfer this volume to a 5 mL polystyrene round-bottom Falcon tube ("FACS tube").
9. Wash the 50 mL Falcon tube with 2 mL of washing solution to recover cells that might have been left in the original tube. Add this volume to the 5 mL Falcon tube containing the rest of the sample transferred.
10. Centrifuge at 540 × *g* for 5 min and remove the supernatant by decanting. In case multiple 50 mL tubes were used (because it

was needed to lyse large sample volumes) the cell suspensions from the same sample should be combined at this moment. If the remaining cell volume is lower than 200 μL, washing solution must be added to reach that volume.

3.4 BM and PB Sample Staining

1. Prepare in one tube a mix of the common antibodies from both tubes: 12 μL of CD38ME-FITC + 4 μL of CD56-PE + 20 μL of CD45 PerCP-Cy5.5 + 10 μL of CD19-PE-Cy7 + 4 μL of CD138-BV421 + 20 μL of CD27-BV510.
2. Pipette 200 μL of Bulk lysed sample (with at least 2×10^6 cells) into the tube and mix well.
3. Divide the volume in two different labeled FACS tubes.
4. Add 5 μL of CD117-APC, 6 μL of CD81 APCC750 antibodies and 54 μL of washing solution to the tube 1 and 65 μL of PBS to the tube 2.
5. Mix well and incubate both tubes for 30 min at room temperature, protected from light.
6. Add 100 μL of Reagent A (fixative; Fix&Perm) to each tube, mix thoroughly and incubate for 15 min at room temperature, protected from light.
7. Add 2 mL of washing solution and mix well.
8. Centrifuge for 5 min at 540 × *g*.
9. Discard the supernatant using a vacuum system without disturbing the cell pellet, leaving approximately 100 μL of residual volume. Resuspend the cell pellet by mixing thoroughly.
10. Add 100 μL of Reagent B (permeabilizing solution; Fix&Perm) and mix well.
11. Add 6 μL CD38ME-FITC to tube 1 and 6 μL CD38ME-FITC, 5 μL of KAPPA-APC and 3 μL of LAMBDA-APCC750 to tube 2.
12. Mix well and incubate for 15 min at room temperature, protected from light.
13. Add 2 mL of washing solution and mix well.
14. Centrifuge for 5 min at 540 × *g*.
15. Discard the supernatant using a Pasteur pipette or vacuum system without disturbing the cell pellet, leaving approximately 100 μL of residual volume.
16. Resuspend the cell pellet in 500 μL of 1× PBS.
17. Acquire the entire tubes at medium flow rate after staining or, if it is not immediately acquired, store at 4 °C for 1 h maximum until measured in the flow cytometer. Link the EuroFlow compensation setup before the sample acquisition.

3.5 Definition of Sample Quality

1. Cell viability is assessed by defining the number of total events acquired in the cytometer and the number of nucleated viable cells. Any difference greater than 20% between both indicates a sample with low cell viability.
2. Different markers (e.g., CD38) versus time must be used to assess the quality and continuity of data acquisition, which provides, for example, the opportunity to gate out air bubbles and/or clogs, thus eliminating periods of time of unstable flow (Fig. 5).
3. NGF provides useful information about the composition of the sample, including the potential existence of significant contamination by PB in BM aspirates by the identification of BM-associated cell subsets, (in addition to CD138 normal and mature PCs) such as: CD117hi mast cells, CD38+ CD19+ CD45lo B-cell precursors and CD117+ CD45int myeloid precursors. Samples in which PCs (both normal and clonal), mast cells, and B-cell and myeloid precursors are not detected must be classified as nonrepresentative for MRD assessment. All samples, in which at least two BM-specific cell populations are detected, must be considered suitable for MRD studies since different treatment strategies (e.g., alkylating agents) and/or different treatment stages (e.g., induction vs. stem cell transplantation) may induce depletion of specific BM cell subsets (Fig. 6).

3.6 Plasma Cell Quantitation and Interpretation

The use of initial gates to identify PCs and discriminate them from all other cell populations are drawn generously enough to include as many PCs events as possible, allowing for variants that express lower CD38, CD45, and/or CD138 to be included, while excluding contaminating lymphocytes, doublets and other cellular debris. The recommended gating steps are as follows:

1. Use of light scatter dot plots to exclude doublets, (FSC-Height versus FSC-Area), (SSC-Height vs. SSC-Area) and debris, (SSC-Area vs. FSC-Area) while exercising caution not to exclude, from initial gating, hyperdiploid or tetraploid PCs which exhibit aberrantly high FSC-Area and SSC-Area, but for example low, FSC-Height.
2. Generous gating is then performed to encompass all potential CD38+ and CD138+ PCs (E) which is further refined by incorporating all CD38+ bright events plotted against CD45 (F). CD45 is helpful for gating but should not be used as a marker for cell exclusion since both normal and neoplastic PCs have variable CD45 expression (Fig. 7).
3. Further characterization of plasma cells: albeit heterogeneous, the normal BM PC immunophenotype is highly conserved in normal bone marrow samples, as well as between individual

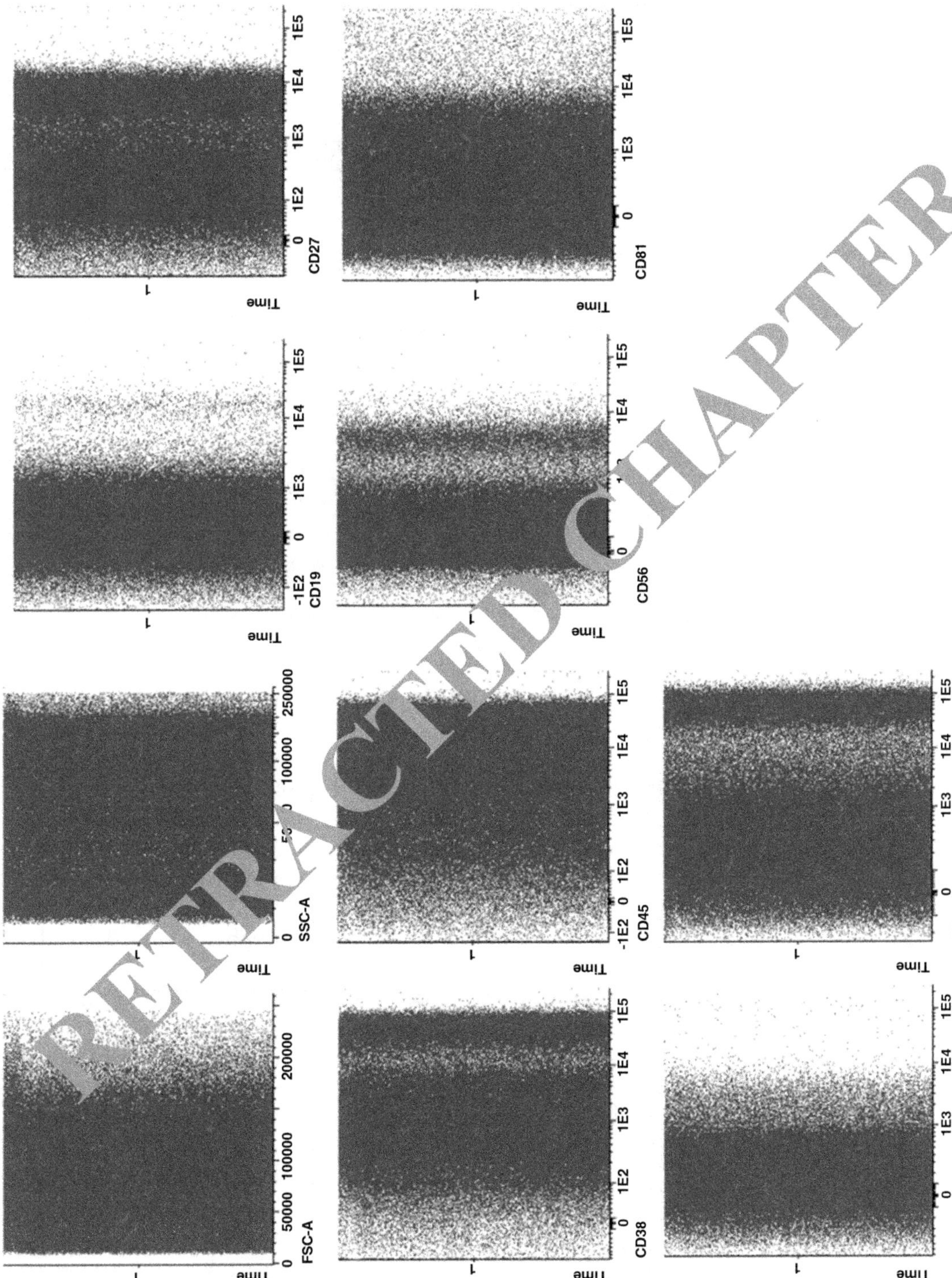

Fig. 5 Dot plots showing different markers versus time to assess the continuity of data acquisition

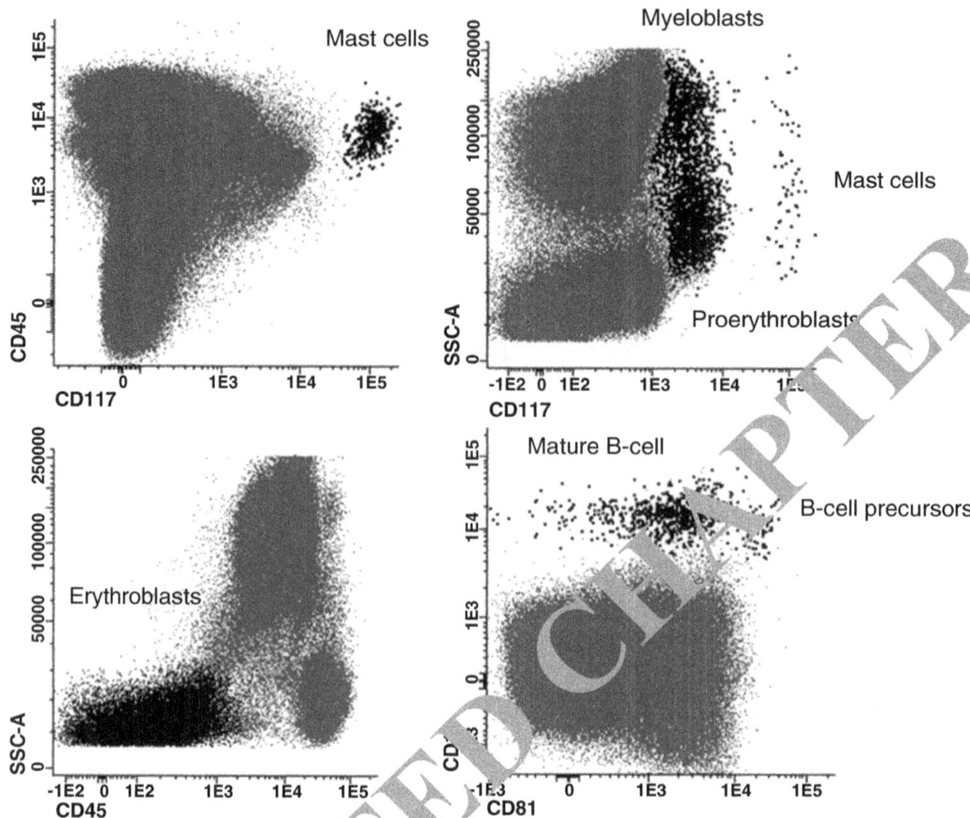

Fig. 6 Identification of BM-associated cell subsets: mast cells, myeloblasts, myeloid precursors, proerythroblasts, and B cell precursors

patient samples at different disease stages, except when antibody-based therapies have been used (e.g., anti-CD38). In this regard, BM PCs from healthy donors, patients with non-plasma cell related diseases, or regenerating BM following chemotherapy in patients with non-PC related diseases, have fully overlapping and highly similar immunophenotypes. In addition, such normal PC immunophenotypes do not overlap with that of >97% of neoplastic PCs from MM patients. That notwithstanding, it should be noted that appropriate multivariate analysis with >6 markers is required to reach such an applicability, because it is now well recognized that minor subsets of normal BM PCs can express some markers with intensity levels previously considered to be aberrant.

Normal PCs show heterogeneous expression of CD19 and CD45, they are usually negative for CD117, and they invariably show homogeneously bright expression of CD81. In turn, CD56 expression is present in a small subset (between 5 and 20%) of normal PCs, the latter plasma cell subset being more frequently found in post-treatment BM samples. Accordingly, normal PCs typically show heterogeneous or bimodal expression for

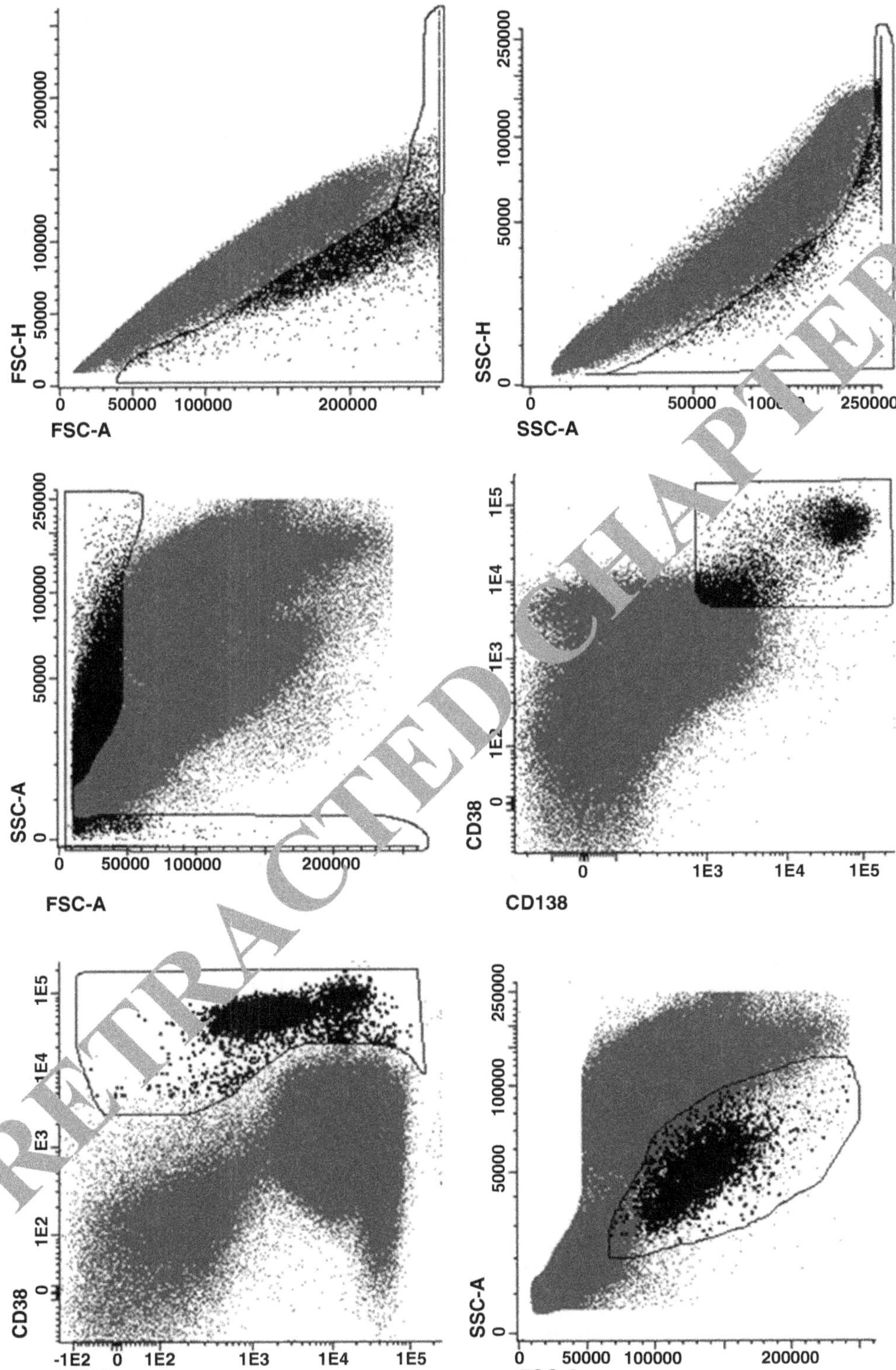

Fig. 7 Gating strategy for identifying the BM PC compartment

some of the most commonly used markers (e.g., CD19, CD45 or CD56) while neoplastic PCs from MM patients usually have more homogeneous antigen expression. Neoplastic PCs might often show additional aberrancies, such as CD117 expression, weaker CD38 expression, and increased FSC and/or SSC features; noteworthy, such aberrancies are coexpressed within the same cell population, whereas immunophenotypic variations in normal PCs tend to be heterogeneous and/or distributed among different well-defined subsets. Provided that a sufficient number of PCs are acquired, analysis of cytoplasmic light chain expression within specific PCs subsets showing myeloma-like aberrant phenotypes (e.g., CD19-negative or CD56-positive plasma cells), is a valuable second step to confirm the normal vs. aberrant nature of such PCs.

4. Defining phenotypically aberrant PCs: no single parameter reliably distinguishes neoplastic PCs from normal PCs; however, even a limited (six colors) combination of antibodies in a single tube can achieve this in virtually all cases providing a sufficient number of cellular events measured in the flow cytometer. Internal positive (e.g., B-cells for CD19 and CD81, NK cells for CD56, myeloid progenitors and mast cells for CD117) and negative control (e.g., erythroblasts for CD45) cell populations represent a highly reliable strategy to define normal vs. aberrant phenotypic expression profiles (Fig. 8).
5. The 2006 Bethesda International Consensus Recommendations advise on the reporting of antigen expression as being reduced, normal or increased in intensity compared to that expressed on appropriate reference cell populations [11]. Reporting in this manner provides a clearer picture of the immunophenotypic deviation from the normal PC immunophenotype and minimizes the impact of variability in reagent and instrument performance between laboratories. Reporting should include the percentage of positive cells for each marker within the specific neoplastic PC compartment. The discrimination between normal PCs and neoplastic PCs on phenotypic grounds has to be multiparametric, i.e., the identification of a neoplastic PC population should never be based on the isolated deviation of a single marker. As described above, analysis of the CyIgκ/CyIgλ plasma cell ratio within specific PC subsets defined on the basis of other surface markers (e.g., CD19− CD45− CD56+) is informative to confirm the clonal vs polyclonal nature of such PC subsets (Fig. 9).
6. The most common immunophenotype of normal PCs could be described as CD38+ bright, CD138+ bright, CD19+, CD45+, CD27+, CD56−, CD81+, CD117−, with a polyclonal CyIgκ/CyIgλ ratio. Minor subsets of normal PCs (typically representing <30% of total normal PCs) exhibit less

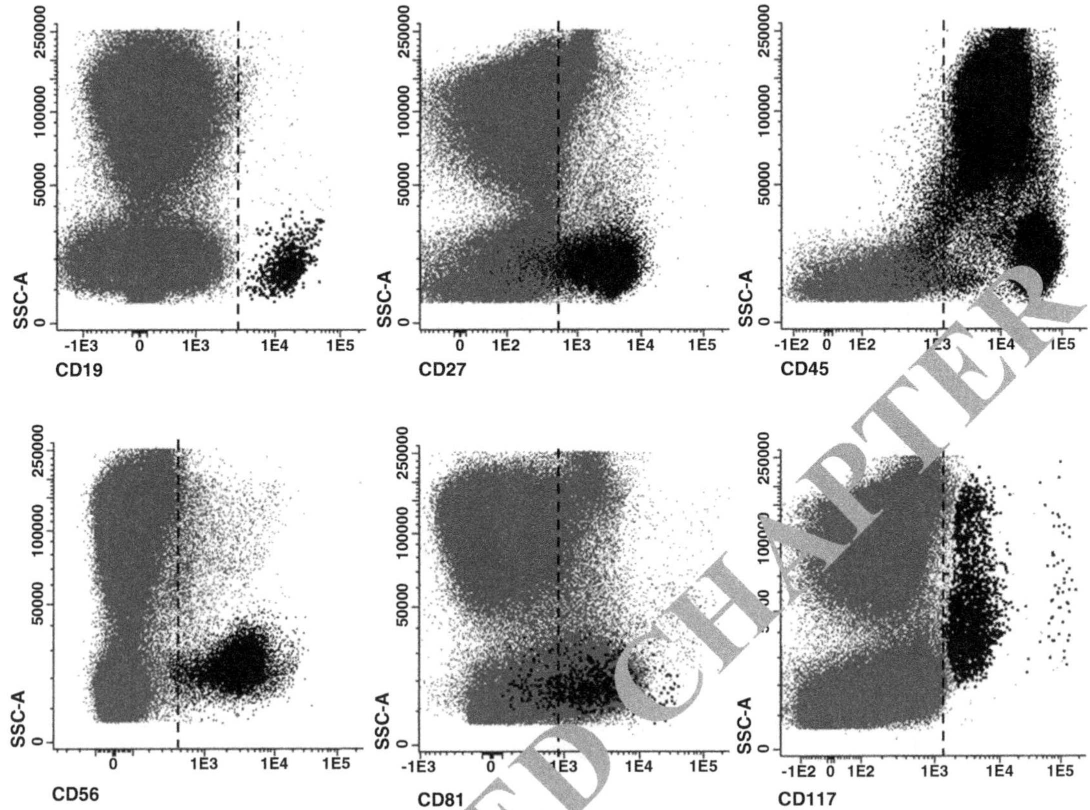

Fig. 8 Expression of routinely used antigens on bone marrow aspirates

"typical" antigen expression patterns such as: CD19−, CD45+/low, CD20+, CD27low, and CD56+. In contrast, neoplastic PCs show aberrant phenotypes consisting of multiple possible combinations of the following aberrant antigenic profiles: CD38low (dimmer than normal PCs), CD19−, CD45−, CD27low, CD56+/bright, CD81−/low, CD117+, in association with monoclonal CyIgκ or CyIgλ expression.

3.7 Reporting a Sample as MRD Positive, MRD Negative, or Unsuitable for MRD Assessment

The guidelines of the International Myeloma Working Group reported in 2016 establish that an MRD negative result is defined when abnormal plasma cells are undetectable at a level of sensitivity of at least 0,001% [12]. However, this is on the proviso that the BM aspirate sample is deemed suitable using the criteria defined earlier, by visualizing all BM cells simultaneously. Thus, the threshold used to distinguish MRD-positive from MRD-negative may vary from sample to sample, and it is recommended to report on the level of MRD and the assay limit of detection in addition to classifying patients as MRD-negative vs. MRD-positive. PC levels should be reported as a percentage from all nucleated cells, since this is likely to offer a better comparison with molecular techniques than reporting as a percentage of leucocytes because DNA is typi-

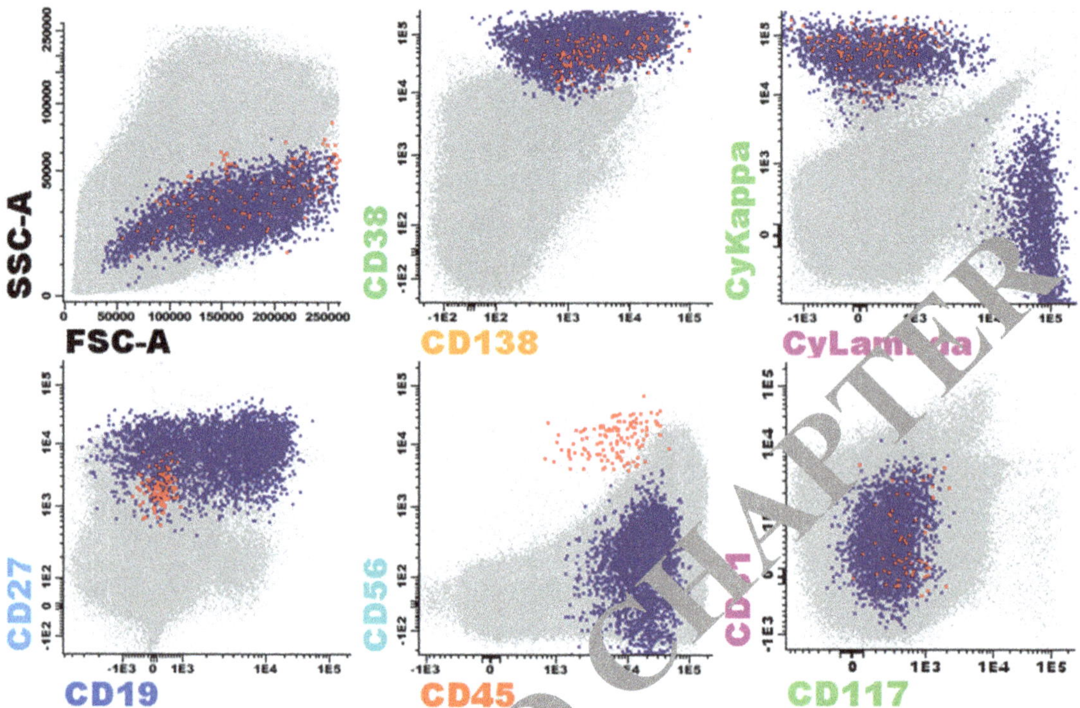

Fig. 9 Normal (in blue) and neoplastic PCs (in red) coexisting within the BM PC compartment

cally isolated from all nucleated cells. Multicenter data has shown that using 0,001%/10^{-5} as the limit of detection for MRD monitoring by flow is of clear prognostic value [13, 14]. Thus, current and future MRD analyses should target a lower limit of detection of 0,0002%/2×10^{-6}, which requires acquisition of at least 1×10^7 bone marrow nucleated cells. The final conclusion of the report should be a categorical assessment (MRD-positive or MRD-negative) of the patients' MRD status, but patient-specific limit of detection (LOD) and limit of quantitation (LOQ) must always be provided. There are numerous studies demonstrating that 20 events are a conservative value for the smallest (homogeneous) population that can be detected in a given flow cytometric list mode data file by experienced operators. This implies that the LOD can be estimated as 100 × 20/total number of nucleated viable single-cells analyzed. Similarly, it is also widely accepted that more than 40 events is a standard threshold for reproducible enumeration of a cell population by experienced flow cytometer operators; consequently, the limit of quantification can be estimated as 100 × 40/total number of nucleated viable single cells analyzed. Thus, the LOD and the LOQ only depend on the total number of cells analyzed.

4 Notes

1. The stock Bulk lysis buffer must be stored in the refrigerator (2–7 °C) for no more than 6 months. The working solution must be stored at room temperature (18–25 °C) for no more than 1 week. pH of both solutions must be stable at 7,4.
2. The pH of the washing buffer is recommended to be set and maintained at 7,4. BSA must have a purity of more than 98%.
3. The peak, that has to be taken as the reference to set PMT voltages, must be indicated on the lot of the 8-peak rainbow beads. Target MFI values vary for different lots and peaks obtained for the 8-peak Rainbow beads may differ from those listed in Table 1. Updated information on lot- and peak-specific target MFI values is also available at the EuroFlow web site [10]. The 8th peak would be the brightest peak and 7th would be the next one downward.
4. For LAMBDA, the fluorophore APCH7 must be selected and "cyLAMBDA" must be written (the same spelling as it is on the experiment layout of the sample acquisition).
5. If there are less than 1.000 events in the positive (P2) gate, repeat recording and "Append" more events to the original recorded tube.
6. Unless otherwise indicated by users, FACSDiVa takes by default as negative reference population for all single stained control tubes, the population gated as "P1" in the unstained control tube.
7. Events under "P2" gates on all the single stained tubes act as the positive reference population for fluorescence compensation.
8. Since both positive and negative reference populations must be of the same "type" (e.g., cells/cells or beads/beads), in CompBeads-containing compensation controls, an additional "P3" gate must be created by users, containing the negative reference bead population (Fig. 3). FACSDiva software will consider these "P3" gated events as the negative reference just for the specific tube it was created.

References

1. Flores-Montero J, Sanoja-Flores L, Paiva B et al (2017) Next generation flow for highly sensitive and standardized detection of minimal residual disease in multiple myeloma. Leukemia 31(10):2094–2103
2. Theunissen P, Mejstrikova E, Sedek L et al (2017) Standardized flow cytometry for highly sensitive MRD measurements in B-cell acute lymphoblastic leukemia. Blood. 129:347–357
3. Kumar S, Paiva B, Anderson KC et al (2016) International Myeloma Working Group consensus criteria for response and minimal residual disease assessment in multiple myeloma. Lancet Oncol 17:e328–e346

4. Kumar S, Rajkumar SV, Kyle RA et al (2005) Prognostic value of circulating plasma cells in monoclonal gammopathy of undetermined significance. J Clin Oncol 23:5668–5674
5. Bianchi G, Kyle RA, Larson DR et al (2013) High levels of peripheral blood circulating plasma cells as a specific risk factor for progression of smoldering multiple myeloma. Leukemia 27:680–685
6. Gonsalves WI, Rajkumar SV, Gupta V et al (2014) Quantification of clonal circulating plasma cells in newly diagnosed multiple myeloma: implications for redefining high-risk myeloma. Leukemia 28:2060–2065
7. Paiva B, Pérez-Andrés M, Vídriales M-B et al (2011) Competition between clonal plasma cells and normal cells for potentially overlapping bone marrow niches is associated with a progressively altered cellular distribution in MGUS vs myeloma. Leukemia 25:697–706
8. Gonsalves WI, Rajkumar SV, Dispenzieri A et al (2017) Quantification of circulating clonal plasma cells via multiparametric flow cytometry identifies patients with smoldering multiple myeloma at high risk of progression. Leukemia 31:130–135
9. CS-T-Application-Guide.pdf. http://trigenotoul.com/wp-content/uploads/2014/12/CS-T-Application-Guide.pdf. 40–47.
10. EuroFlow. https://euroflow.org/usr/pub/pub.php.
11. Wood BL, Arroz M, Barnett D et al (2007) 2006 Bethesda International Consensus recommendations on the immunophenotypic analysis of hematolymphoid neoplasia by flow cytometry: optimal reagents and reporting for the flow cytometric diagnosis of hematopoietic neoplasia. Cytometry B Clin Cytom 72(Suppl 1):S14–S22
12. Rawstron AC, Orfao A, Beksac M et al (2008) Report of the European Myeloma Network on multiparametric flow cytometry in multiple myeloma and related disorders. Haematologica 93:431–438
13. Paiva B, Cedena M-T, Puig N et al (2016) Minimal residual disease monitoring and immune profiling in multiple myeloma in elderly patients. Blood 127:3165–3174
14. Korde N, Roschewski M, Zingone A et al (2015) Treatment with carfilzomib-lenalidomide-dexamethasone with lenalidomide extension in patients with smoldering or newly diagnosed multiple myeloma. JAMA Oncology 1:746–754

Chapter 3

Cytoplasmic Immunoglobulin Vs. DNA Analysis by Flow Cytometry

Daisy Alapat

Abstract

Cytoplasmic immunoglobulin (CIg) vs DNA by flow cytometric (FCM) method allows us to detect DNA content of the neoplastic plasma cells with monotypic cytoplasmic immunoglobulin and also provide us with clear distinction from normal polytypic plasma cells. Abnormalities in cellular DNA content (DNA aneuploidy) and cell cycle determination (proliferative activity) can be measured rapidly by flow cytometry. FCM can measure gross differences in DNA content and distinguish a cell population with normal DNA content, or diploid from a cell population with an abnormal or aneuploid DNA content. With the dual parameter procedure a monoclonal plasma cell population can be identified down to less than 0.1–0.05% of all cells.

Key words DNA Index, Cytoplasmic immunoglobulin, Kappa and lambda, cIg/DNA

1 Introduction

Cells in different stages of the cell cycle have different but predictable amounts of DNA. Normal cells have one set of chromosomes or a diploid DNA content. The terminology for this by FCM is a normal DNA Index (DI) of 1. The majority (>95%) of normal cells are quiescent cells and are in G0 stage of the cell cycle. The G0 cells enter the G1 phase in which enzymes needed for synthesis are produced. From G1 phase, cells enter into DNA synthesis phase called S phase. The S phase contains cells with a continuous varying amount of DNA (Fig. 1). The cells then enter the G2 phase where specialized proteins and RNA are synthesized. The G2 phase then terminates in mitotic division or the M phase. G2/M cells now have two sets of chromosomes or twice the amount of DNA of G0/1 phase. The S phase fraction of most normal cells is less than 5%. By determining the S phase % of tumors, the proliferation activity of the tumor cells can be

Christoph Heuck and Niels Weinhold (eds.), *Multiple Myeloma: Methods and Protocols*, Methods in Molecular Biology, vol. 1792, https://doi.org/10.1007/978-1-4939-7865-6_3,

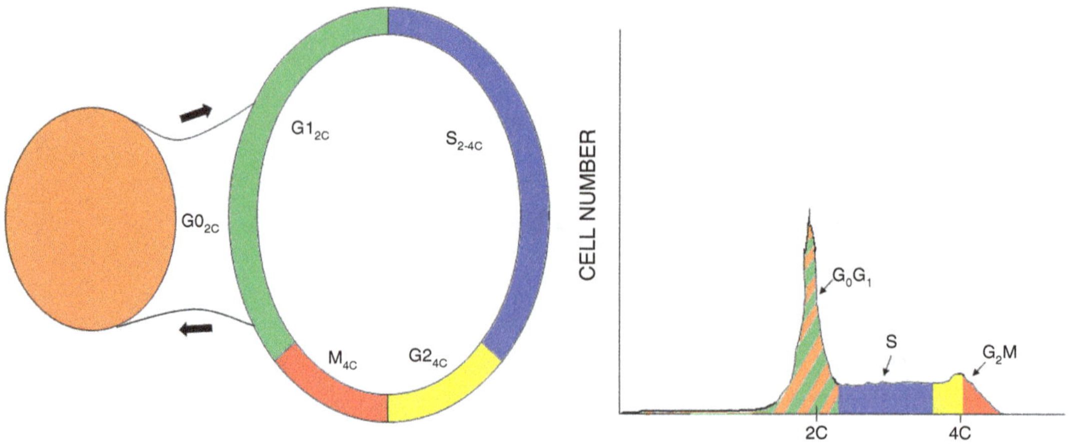

Fig. 1 Relationship between cell cycle phases and DNA histogram

estimated, and cell cycle specific drugs may be more optimally used in treatment. By comparing the amount of DNA in the G0/1 peak of tumor cells to a normal diploid G0/1 peak, the degree of ploidy or abnormal amount of DNA may be determined. This is expressed as DI. The normal G0/1 peak is given the designation of diploid with an index of 1.0 [1, 2].

The plasma cells of patients with multiple myeloma usually contain an abnormal DNA and an increased RNA content, permitting the quantitation of plasma cells by flow cytometry [3, 4]. A typical feature of plasma cells is the presence of cytoplasmic immunoglobulin (CIg). Approximately 80% plasma cell myeloma patients have an abnormal DNA stem line with 10–15% more DNA than normal hematopoietic cells. In addition, cytoplasmic RNA content is markedly increased in all myeloma patients that are producing cytoplasmic immunoglobulin. Flow cytometric analysis of monotypic CIg and DNA content of bone marrow cells from patients with multiple myeloma patients allows S-phase determination of the CIg(+) plasma cells separately from the Clg(−) hematopoietic cell pool [5, 6]. Examples for histograms of normal diploid cells without light chain restriction and kappa-positive aneuploidy myeloma cells are shown in Figs. 2 and 3, respectively.

The DI is the ratio of the mode or mean of the relative DNA content of the G0/1 cells of the sample divided by the mode or mean of the relative DNA measurement of the diploid G0/1 cells. The diagnosis of DNA aneuploidy (abnormal DNA content) should be reported only when at least two separate G0/1 peaks are demonstrated [7].

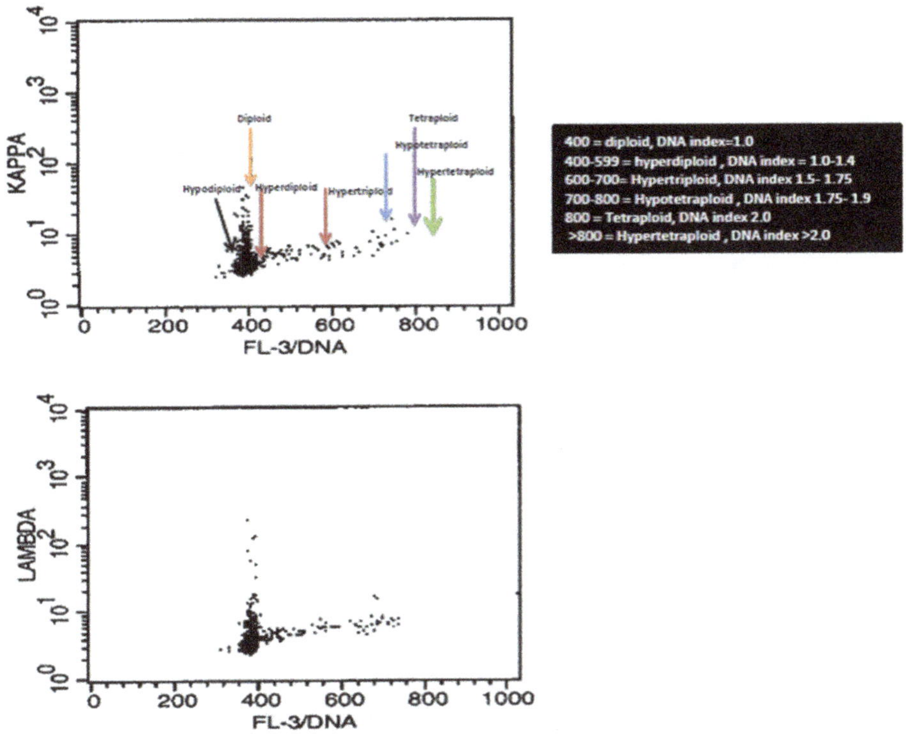

Fig. 2 Histogram of Normal diploid without light chain restriction highlighting regions by hypoploid, diploid, hyperdiploid, triploid, hypotetraploid, tetraploid, and hypertetraploid

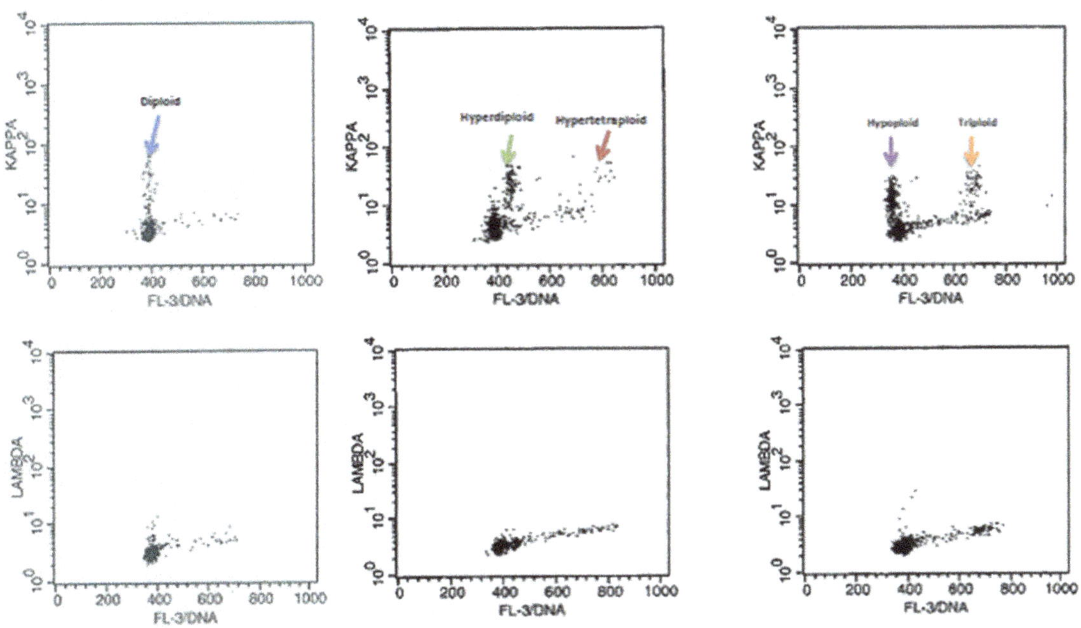

Fig. 3 Sample histograms of diploid, hyperdiploid, triploid, and hypertetraploid stem lines

2 Materials

Specimen	Requirement	Storage	Rejection
Peripheral blood	Na heparin	RT	Clotted
Bone marrow	Na heparin	RT	Clotted
Body fluids	Fresh	RT	Clotted
Solid tissue, FNA	Fresh/in RPMI	RT	Necrotic

2.1 Equipment

1. FACScan Flow Cytometer.
2. Cell quest software program.

2.1.1 Reagents

1. 10× Stock propidium iodide (PI): Add 100 mg (0.10 g) P1 to 200 mL of PBS. Mix for 10–15 min. Filter through a 0.2 μm filter. Place solution in foil-wrapped bottle to protect from light. Label, date, and store at 4 °C (6 months expiration date) (*see* **Notes 1** and **2**).
2. 10× stock ribonuclease A: 100 mg (in X amount of liquid for each lot) up to 10 mL PBS. Measure the total volume in the vial and dilute up to 10 mL pH to 7.4 with 6–7 drops of 1 M NaOH. Aliquot 10× in 100 μL amounts and freeze at −20 °C (1 year expiration date) (*see* **Note 2**).
3. 1× working RNase: thaw 10× RNase and dilute 1:10 with PBS. Working solution concentration is 1 mg/mL. Final sample concentration will be 0.1 mg/mL for 100 μL per sample. Store at 4 °C (1 week expiration).
4. 95% ethanol stored at −20 °C.
5. RPMI Holding Media: 100 mL RPMI 1640 Media w/20 mM HEPES and L-glutamine w/o $NaHCO_3$), add 0.5 mL gentamycin sulfate (10 mg/mL stock), 2 mL penicillin 5000 U/mL streptomycin 5 mg/mL, 5 mL fetal calf serum (FCS), and 2 mL heparin (100 USP/mL stock)
6. PBS without sodium azide: dissolve Dulbecco's Phosphate Buffered Saline powder contents of 1 l bottle in 1 l of distilled H_2O. Mix well and adjust pH to 7.4. Store at 4 °C.
7. Heat inactivated fetal calf serum (FCS)
8. 2% FCS in PBS (2% PBS): add 2 mL FCS to 98 mL PBS (30 day expiration date).
9. Ammonium Chloride (NH4CL) Lyse Solution for RBC: For 250 mL combine 2.065 g NH_4CL, 0.25 g $KHCO_3$, and 9.25 mg EDTA in a 50 mL tube. Transfer reagents to graduated cylinder and add 250 mL dH_2O. Rinse out 50 mL reagent tube with water and add the rinse to the cylinder. Mix 15 min. Check pH and use when pH has stabilized at 7.4 (*see* **Note 3**).

10. Ficoll-Paque. Store at room temperature (opened bottles are stored at 4 °C).
11. Anti-Kappa $_{\text{fitc}}$ F(AB)$_2$ polyclonal: use 100 μL at 1:200 dilution. Dilute in 1× PBS (stable for 1 week) (*see* **Note 2**).
12. Anti-Lambda $_{\text{fitc}}$ F(AB)$_2$ polyclonal: use 100 μL at 1:200 dilution. Dilute in 1× PBS (stable for 1 week) (*see* **Note 2**).
13. Positive kappa/lambda controls (store at −20 °C).
14. DNA Check Beads: Add 5–8 drops of well-mixed beads to 0.5 mL of 1× PBS (stable for 1 week).
15. Alcohol fixed Chicken Red Blood Cells (CRBC)
    (a) Prepare the wash buffer by mixing 9 g NaCl and 0.33 g anhydrous $CaCI_2$ in 1 l H_2O.
    (b) To prepare saponin solution add 25 mg saponin powder to 50 mL of wash buffer (*see* **Note 4**).
    (c) Wash 5.0 mL of heparinized CRBC in 50 mL wash buffer to remove plasma. Wash a minimum of 3 times in 50 mL tubes. Centrifuge at 400 × *g* for 15 min.
    (d) Add 20–25 mL of saponin solution to CRBC pellet and mix well: Rock tube for 10 min at room temperature. Partial but not complete clearing may be seen as cells lyse.
    (e) Centrifuge lysate at 400 × *g* for 10 min. Aspirate supernatant and resuspend pellet in 15 mL of wash buffer. Repeat washes until all traces of red are gone. A small pellet of unlysed RBC may be seen. Carefully remove the unlysed clump with a Pasteur pipette.
    (f) After final centrifugation add 10–25 mL of cold wash buffer. Disperse thoroughly with syringe and 21 g needle.
    (g) Fix cells while vortexing by rapidly adding an equal amount of ice-cold absolute EtoH.
    (h) Store fixed nuclei in the refrigerator. CEN will settle out over time and may need syringing or sonicating before use. Clumping gradually increases over time. Adjust concentration so as to use 5–10 μL per tube.
16. Diploid ethanol fixed cells: use as diploid control and in admixture studies when needed. Use previously fixed normal bloods or mononuclear product.

3 Methods

3.1 Ficoll Procedure (*See* Note 5)

1. Blood: dilute 4 mL blood with 4 mL 1× PBS. Bone marrow: dilute 3 mL bone marrow with 5 mL 1× PBS.
2. Pipette 3 mL of Ficoll-Paque (F-P) into a labeled 15 mL conical-shaped tube and overlay 4 mL of diluted sample onto

it. Layer two tubes per 8 mL of diluted sample. Do not mix F-P and blood interface while layering as this will make a poor separation.

3. Centrifuge layered sample at 568 × *g* for 30 min at room temperature. Be sure the brake is turned off.
4. After centrifugation, aspirate the clear upper supernatant from each tube. Remove the cloudy band of mononuclear cells from both tubes and pool together in a clean labeled tube containing 5 mL PBS. Pipette up and down several times to mix sample in the final tube. Do not invert tubes to mix. Minimize the amount of extra solution you take from around the mononuclear layer as either serum or Ficoll will contaminate the cell suspension.
5. Centrifuge at 169 × *g* for 7 min at room temperature.
6. Remove supernatant from cell pellet, leaving less than 0.5 mL. Resuspend the cell pellet by gently raking the centrifuge tube across the top of a test tube rack. If cell pellets appear bloody add 2–3 mL of NH_4Cl (*see* **Note 6**). Add 1 mL to tubes with low cell recovery based on cell pellet size.
7. Centrifuge at 169 × *g* for 7 min.
8. Remove lysed supernatant and shake cell pellets to resuspend. Add 2 mL of 1× PBS to each tube. Add 1 mL to tubes with low cell recovery based on cell pellet size.
9. Centrifuge at 169 × *g* for 7 min at room temperature.
10. Remove supernatant and resuspend the cell pellet by gently raking the centrifuge tube across the top of a test tube rack. Add 1 mL of PBS to all tubes. Add 2 mL PBS to tubes with large cell pellets and 0.5 mL PBS to tubes with very small cell pellets. Gently raking the centrifuge tube across the top of a test tube rack to resuspend cells.
11. Perform cell count for all specimens. Mix any specimen with clumps. Cell counts less than 5×10^5 should be diluted in 0.5 mL 1× PBS. Cell counts from $2–9.5 \times 10^6$ should be diluted in 1 mL 1× PBS. Any specimen with $>1 \times 10^7$ to 2×10^7 cells/mL should be diluted into 2 mL 1× PBS. Remove extra cells and dilute remaining specimen up to 2 mL 1× PBS total. Record the count according to total cell count of remaining cells in 2 mL.
12. Remove ETOH from freezer to fix cells. While vortexing the tube, add appropriate amount of ice-cold ETOH to each specimen. Add ETOH drop wise while cells are mixing. Do not add the ETOH in all at once. This will cause clumping (*see* **Notes 7** and **8**).
    (a) 1 mL of cells—add 2.8 mL of 95% ETOH.

(b) 2 mL of cells—add 5.6 mL of 95% ETOH.

(c) 0.5 mL of cells—add 1.4 of 95% ETOH.

13. Place fixed specimens in refrigerator (4 °C–8 °C) (*see* **Note 9**).

3.2 CIg Vs DNA Staining Procedure

1. Place 2 × 10^6–4 × 10^6 ETOH fixed cells into labeled 5 mL Falcon plastic tubes. Centrifuge at 169 × *g* for 5 min. Decant supernatant and mix cell pellet by raking the bottom of the tubes across a rack (*see* **Note 10**).
2. Resuspend cell pellets in 1 mL of 1× PBS and count cells, if needed. Use 1 × 10^6 to 2 × 10^6 cells per tube. Split each sample between the two 5 mL tubes labeled kappa and lambda.
3. Spin at 169 × *g* for 5 min. Decant all of the supernatant.
4. Add 100 μL of the diluted light chain antibodies. Mix gently. Incubate 30 min at 40 °C in the dark.
5. Add 2 mL of PBS and centrifuge at 169 × *g* @ 4 °C for 7 min. Remove all supernatant from pellet. Resuspend cells by raking the bottom of the tubes across a rack.
6. Add 0.4 mL 1× PBS, 100 μL 1× RNase, and 40 μL of 10× PI to the cell pellets. Mix gently.
7. Incubate tubes at room temperature for 10 min in the dark. Analyze within 2 h. Filter each sample through 25 μm mesh immediately before analysis to remove cell clumps.

3.3 Sample Acquisition (See Note 11)

1. Turn on the FACScan. The fluid control knob should be set on STANDBY. Warm up time for the laser is 5 min. During this time the NOT READY light is on. After 5 min, the STANDBY light comes on.
2. Turn on the computers from the startup button on the hard drive.
3. Check Fluid Containers:
   (a) Sheath reservoir should be no more than 3/4 full.
   (b) Waste container should be empty.
   (c) Switch Vent Valve to UP position to pressurize.
4. Move the Droplet Containment Module (DCM) arm to the right.
5. Place a fresh tube of filtered deionized H_2O (DI water) on sample injection port (SIP) and prime the instrument by switching to RUN mode for a few minutes. Place in STANDBY position until ready to acquire samples.
6. Open the Cell Quest software program.
7. Use DNA Check beads to check whether the instrument is maintaining a constant mean channel from a constant PMT setting over time. A low bead CV is important in establishing

the resolution of the instrument. A CV of less than three for beads, on FL 2 or 3 PMT is needed to ensure good resolution for sample G0/1 peaks (*see* **Note 12**).

8. Mix first sample and run sample setup mode to make any minor adjustments in FL3 or FL2 peaks or FL1 vs FL3 dot plot. Adjust diploid G0/1 population to channel 400 in FL-3/orange and channel 200 in FL-2/red histograms. Adjust the negative light chain green FL to just below the 1st decade in the FL1 vs FL3 dot plot.
9. Run each specimen set starting with the Kappa and ending with the Lambda tube. Acquire 5000 events in each tube.
10. Positive kappa and lambda controls are included in each run.
11. After acquisition, clean with filtered 10% bleach for 10 min then filtered water for 10 min.

3.4 Sample Analysis

1. Pull the 2 files to be analyzed, starting with Kappa vs DNA in the top dot plot and Lambda vs DNA in the second dot plot (Fig. 4, *see* **Note 13**).
2. Adjust boxes for each sample as needed. Set boxes around the light chain negative G0/1 and S/G2M populations and the positive light chain cell cycle populations. The % for the light chain population is determined for each light chain and any excess is established. Use the additional boxes for the cell cycle of any aneuploid populations.
3. Print dotplots with numbers and perform calculations.
4. To calculate the DNA Index divide FL-3 X-axis mean channel of the light chain positive G0/1 population by the X-axis mean channel of the main G0/1 light chain negative population. If the tumor peak is lower than 1.0 it is called hypodiploid; if it is greater than 1.0 it is called hyperdiploid (>1.0–1.5), triploid (>1.5–2.0) or tetraploid (>2.0) based on DI number. All of these cases are considered aneuploidy (*see* **Note 14**).
5. To calculate the Cytoplasmic Intrinsic index divide the Y mean channel of light chain positive G0/I by the Y mean channel of diploid G0/I negative cells (*see* **Note 15**).
6. To calculate the % cell cycle of each phase use the following equation: (number of events in each cycle region)/(total number of events) × 100.
7. To calculate the +light chain population use the following equation: (number of events for the light chain positive population)/(total number of events) × 100.

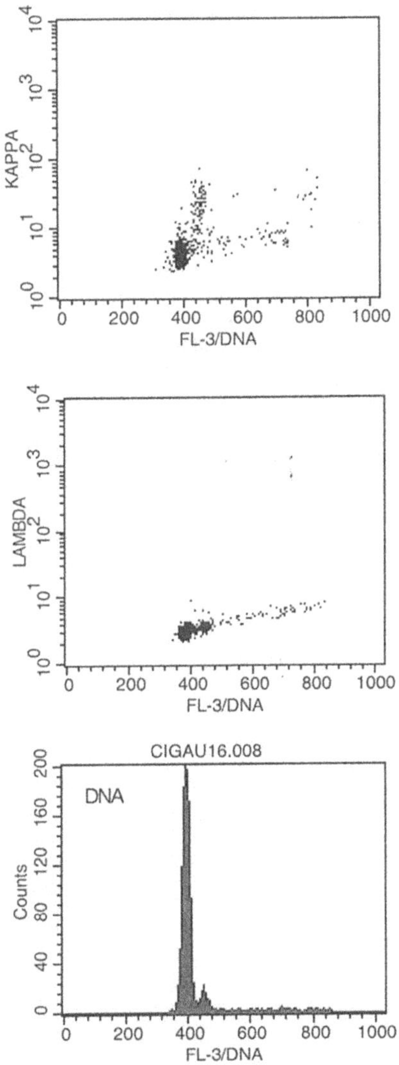

Cytoplasmic Immunoglobulin/DNA Analysis

	% Positive Light Chain	DNA Index (DI)	CIg Index* (CI)
KAPPA diploid	<1	1.0	
aneuploid 1	6	1.16	5.0
aneuploid 2	<1	2.07	8.9
LAMBDA diploid	<1	1.0	
aneuploid 1			
aneuploid 2			

DNA Cell Cycle Analysis

Overall Cell Cycle:	%G0/1	%S + G2/M
diploid	89	5
aneuploid 1	6	
aneuploid 2		

Normal range: No light chain excess. DNA INDEX = 1.0
* CI = Ratio of Intensity of CIg+ cells/ CIg- cells.

DIAGNOSIS FOR CYTOPLASMIC Ig/DNA:

DI = 1.0, 1.16, 2.07 ; % S = 5 ; CIg Index = 5.0, 8.9

Hyperdiploid and hypertetraploid with kappa light chain excess in 6% of all cells with a Cig index of 5.0 and 8.9.

Fig. 4 Sample of final report: Myeloma patient showing hyperdiploid and hypertetraploid stem lines with kappa light chain excess

4 Notes

1. Propidium iodide is a possible carcinogen, so be cautious. PI is light sensitive.
2. New lots of PI, RNase, and light chain antibodies are titrated on cell populations using a three or four point dilution range. The G0/1 peak or the positive LC cell population is gated and

the mean channel and % positive is recorded. The concentration with the highest mean channel, the highest % positive cells and which has the highest separation from the negative population is used.

3. Lysis buffer should be made freshly daily.
4. Saponin powder is poisonous. Do not inhale. Handle with care.
5. Perform all steps at room temperature.
6. Minor contaminant of red blood cells does not need to be removed. Do not lyse tissue more than twice as this increases the nucleated cells cellular debris.
7. Clumpy specimens should be passed through a mesh before they are fixed in alcohol. The alcohol step will maintain the cells in clumps which contribute to a false increase in the G2/M stage and background. A second mesh stage to decrease clumps is performed at the instrument immediately before acquisition.
8. Alcohol fixation can cause cell loss.
9. ETOH fixed cells are stable for years.
10. Do not vortex fixed cells at any stage.
11. Perform instrument calibration and QC steps on a daily to monthly schedule based on the manufacturer's suggestions provided in the manual. This ensures adequate review of the daily characteristics and functions of the instrument and its parts.
12. Settings for new lot numbers of beads are established after a consistent run for a week. Although bead QC is important, sample rejection is based on the quality of sample G0/1 CV only. Beads may have borderline CVs or above 3.0 while samples are still valid to report based on their individual CV.
13. Acquisition of less than 500 events in dot plots may not give reliable results. Unless a distinct pattern of light chain positive events are identified the results should be considered unacceptable.
14. CIg vs DNA Assay sensitivity is 0.1% events for diploid cells with bright light chain positivity and about 0.05% for aneuploid cell populations.
15. In the cases where cIg results are difficult to interpret due to increased back ground light chain expression, investigate slides, cytospins, or CRBC data to help in making a conclusion on cell types in the specimen that may contribute to high background.

References

1. Bauer KD, Clevenger CV, Endow RK et al (1986) Simultaneous nuclear antigen and DNA content quantitation using paraffin-embedded colonic tissue and multiparameter flow cytometry. Cancer Res 46:2428–2434
2. Barlogie B, Alexanian R, Pershouse M et al (1985) Cytoplasmic immunoglobulin content in multiple myeloma. J Clin Invest 76:765–769. https://doi.org/10.1172/JCI112033
3. San Miguel JF, García-Sanz R, González M, Orfão A (1996) DNA cell content studies in multiple myeloma. Leuk Lymphoma 23:33–41. https://doi.org/10.3109/10428199609054799
4. Chan CS, Wormsley SB, Peter JB, Schechter GP (1989) Dual parameter analysis of myeloma cells by flow cytometry. DNA content of cells containing monotypic cytoplasmic immunoglobulin. Am J Clin Pathol 91:12–17
5. Barlogie B, Alexanian R, Gehan EA et al (1983) Marrow cytometry and prognosis in myeloma. J Clin Invest 72:853–861. https://doi.org/10.1172/JCI111056
6. Barlogie B, Alexanian R, Dixon D et al (1985) Prognostic implications of tumor cell DNA and RNA content in multiple myeloma. Blood 66:338–341
7. Hiddemann W, Schumann J, Andreef M et al (1984) Convention on nomenclature for DNA cytometry. Committee on Nomenclature, Society for Analytical Cytology. Cancer Genet Cytogenet 13:181–183

Chapter 4

Deep Profiling of the Immune System of Multiple Myeloma Patients Using Cytometry by Time-of-Flight (CyTOF)

Tina Smets, Frederik Stevenaert, HC Adams 3rd, and Greet Vanhoof

Abstract

Mass cytometry has emerged as a new state-of-the-art technology that enables in-depth characterization of cellular populations and functions at a single cell resolution. We describe the application of this technology to deeply phenotype the blood and bone marrow components of multiple myeloma patients in a clinical setting. This technology allows for simultaneous quantification of more than 40 markers, overcoming the challenges of traditional fluorescence-based flow cytometry.

Key words Mass cytometry, CyTOF, Multiple myeloma, Immunophenotyping, Single cell, Barcoding, Smart tube, Peripheral blood, Bone marrow

1 Introduction

CyTOF (Cytometry by Time-of-Flight) [1, 2] combines cytometry at a single cell level with mass spectrometry. Mass cytometry overcomes the challenges of flow cytometry by using heavy metal ion tags rather than fluorochromes conjugated to antibodies, enabling readout by time-of-flight mass spectrometry. This allows for the combination of many more antibody specificities in single samples without significant spillover between channels, and augments the ability of cytometry to deeply profile immune systems. We applied CyTOF to evaluate an expanded immunophenotyping panel in clinical samples of multiple myeloma patients to determine treatment effects on immune cell subpopulations.

Whole blood and bone marrow samples were collected from patients enrolled in daratumumab clinical studies [3–5]. The Smart Tube™ system was introduced for fixation and storage of patient samples. Samples were tested on CyTOF to analyze baseline immune profiles of patients, as well as treatment effects [6].

The original version of this chapter was revised. The correction to this chapter is available at https://doi.org/10.1007/978-1-4939-7865-6_17

Christoph Heuck and Niels Weinhold (eds.), *Multiple Myeloma: Methods and Protocols*, Methods in Molecular Biology, vol. 1792, https://doi.org/10.1007/978-1-4939-7865-6_4, © Springer Science+Business Media, LLC, part of Springer Nature 2018

2 Materials

Prepare all reagents using ultrapure and analytical grade reagents to avoid any metal contamination. Store all reagents at 4 °C (unless indicated otherwise). All centrifugation steps are performed at 600 × *g* for 6 min at 20 °C.

2.1 Sample Collection

1. Whole blood and bone marrow samples of multiple myeloma patients.
2. Smart Tubes™ (SMART TUBE Inc.).

2.2 Immunophenotyping Antibody Panel

1. Metal conjugated antibodies.
2. Purified antibodies (*see* **Note 1**).
3. MaxPar® Antibody labeling kit (Fluidigm).

2.3 Staining

1. Dulbecco's Phosphate buffered saline without calcium chloride and magnesium chloride (PBS).
2. Stain buffer (BSA) (SB) (BD Biosciences).
3. Water (minimal contamination with heavy metals to avoid interference with mass cytometry analysis).
4. Phosflow Perm Buffer III (BD Biosciences).
5. Perm/wash buffer (10×) (BD Biosciences), dilute in ultrapure water.
6. Thaw/lyse buffer (1000×) (SMART TUBE Inc.), dilute in ultrapure water.
7. Lysis buffer 2 (5×) (SMART TUBE Inc.), dilute stock solution with ultrapure water.
8. Human TruStain FcX (BioLegend).
9. Round bottom FACS tube (5 mL).
10. Conical centrifuge tubes (50 mL).
11. Cell strainer (40 μm).
12. Cooling water bath.
13. Manual counting chamber slides.

2.4 Sample Acquisition on CyTOF

1. Tuning solution (Fluidigm).
2. EQ™ Four Element Calibration Beads (Fluidigm).
3. Wash solution (Fluidigm).
4. Ultrapure water (Fluidigm).
5. Intercalator-Iridium (500 μM) (Fluidigm).
6. 20-Plex Pd Barcoding kit (Fluidigm).
7. Super Sampler.

8. Chiller.
9. CyTOF Mass Cytometer (CyTOF2-Upgrade) (Fluidigm).

2.5 Data Processing

1. CyTOF Software 6. 5.358 for Stand-Alone Processing Workstations (Fluidigm).

3 Methods

3.1 Sample Collection

1. Whole blood and bone marrow samples are collected at the clinical sites, shipped to the central lab, and stored in Smart Tubes until ready for testing. Smart Tubes are used for fixation and storage of the samples.
2. Transfer 1 mL of sample to a Smart Tube, close the tube and break the glass tube inside. Gently mix the tube and incubate at room temperature for 10 min.
3. After fixation, transfer the Smart Tube to a −80 °C freezer for long-term storage (*see* **Note 2**).

3.2 Preparing and Staining Whole Blood Samples

1. Thaw Smart Tubes in a cooling water bath at 10 °C for 20 min, shake gently every 5 min.
2. For each sample, add 20 mL of thaw/lyse buffer to a 50 mL centrifuge tube and place a cell strainer on top. After thawing of the sample, add 2 mL of thaw/lyse buffer to the Smart Tube, mix gently, decant the sample onto the cell strainer.
3. Wash the Smart Tube twice with an additional 3 mL of thaw/lyse buffer. Incubate the sample for 10 min at room temperature. Centrifuge, remove the supernatant and resuspend the cell pellet in 10 mL thaw/lyse buffer, add thaw/lyse buffer to a final volume of 25 mL. Incubate the sample for 10 min at room temperature. Centrifuge, remove the supernatant.
4. If the cell pellet is free of red blood cells (RBC), continue with a washing step with 20 mL of 1× PBS. If the cell pellet contains RBC, an additional lysis step is performed with 20 mL of lysis buffer 2, 10 min incubation at room temperature. Centrifuge, remove the supernatant and resuspend the cell pellet in 10 mL SB.
5. Centrifuge, remove the supernatant and resuspend the cells in 1 mL SB, and count the cells. Keep the cells at 4 °C on ice during counting.
6. Bring 2×10^6 cells in a FACS tube, add SB up to 3 mL, centrifuge and remove supernatant.
7. Add 10 μL of Human TruStain FcX and incubate for 15 min at 4 °C on ice.

8. The mix of metal tagged antibodies that is used for extracellular staining is made in SB to a predetermined optimal concentration. Fifty microliters of this extracellular antibody panel mixture is added to the sample and incubated for at least 30 min at 4 °C on ice (*see* **Note 3**).
9. Add 2 mL of SB and centrifuge, remove supernatant and repeat once.
10. Loosen the cell pellet and add 1 mL of Perm/wash buffer dropwise on a vortex to the cells. Incubate for 15 min at 4 °C on ice. Centrifuge and remove the supernatant.
11. Make a mix of the metal tagged antibodies that are used for intracellular staining to a predetermined optimal concentration in perm/wash buffer. Add 50 μL the intracellular antibody panel mixture to the sample and incubate for at least 30 min at 4 °C on ice (*see* **Note 4**).
12. Add 2 mL of perm/wash buffer and centrifuge, remove supernatant and repeat once.
13. Add 2 mL of SB and centrifuge, remove supernatant.
14. Loosen the cell pellet and add 1 mL of ice-cold perm III buffer dropwise on a vortex to the cells. Incubate for 20 min at 4 °C on ice. From this step the sample can be stored at −80 °C until acquisition on CyTOF.

3.3 Acquisition of Samples on CyTOF

1. Set up the instrument, perform a daily quality control by checking the instrument performance, monitoring the background and tuning the system, according to the manufacturer's instruction.
2. Add 2 mL of SB to the samples in Perm III buffer, centrifuge, and remove supernatant.
3. Add 2 mL of PBS and centrifuge, remove supernatant.
4. Barcoding of the samples. Take the desired barcodes out of the freezer. Add 100 μL of PBS to each barcode (*see* **Note 5**).
5. Resuspend the samples in 800 μL PBS containing Iridium, final concentration 0.25 μM (*see* **Note 6**).
6. Add the diluted barcode to the sample and mix gently. Incubate for 30 min at 4 °C on ice.
7. Add 2 mL of SB and centrifuge, remove supernatant and repeat once.
8. Add 2 mL of ultrapure water and centrifuge, remove supernatant.
9. Resuspend the sample in ultrapure water containing EQ™ Four Element Calibration Beads (1/10), pool all the barcoded samples and run on CyTOF.

3.4 Data Processing

1. After sample acquisition on CyTOF an FCS file is generated that is normalized to allow comparison of data within and across experiments. Normalization of the sample is done with EQ™ Four Element Calibration Beads, which contain natural abundance Cerium (140/142Ce), Europium (151/153Eu), Holmium (165Ho), and Lutetium (175/176Lu). This method normalizes data to a global standard determined for each lot of manufactured EQ Beads, and allows normalization of data within and across experiments. Normalization is performed using CyTOF Software 6. 5.358 for Stand-Alone Processing Workstations.
2. After normalization, the data are debarcoded to deconvolute the different events per barcoded sample. The debarcoder assigns each event to its original barcode consisting of a specific pattern of the different Palladium (102/104/105/106/108/110 Pd) isotopes. Separate FCS files are generated for each barcoded sample allowing further analysis per sample.
3. FCS files are uploaded in CytoBankTM software for manual gating and SPADE (spanning-tree progression of density-normalized events) analysis (Fig. 1) [7].

4 Notes

1. For the antibody panel metal conjugated antibodies commercially available from Fluidigm (CD11b_144Nd, CD4_145Nd, CD8_146Nd, CD34_148Nd, CD45RO_149Sm, CD27_155Gd, CD137_158Gd, CD11c_162Dy, CD15_164Dy, CD274_175Lu, CD16_209Bi, CD45_89Y) and purified antibodies labeled in-house with the MaxPar® Antibody labeling kit (CD66b_139La, Active Caspase-3_141Pr, CD20_142Nd, CD3_143Nd, CD24_147Sm, CD138_150Nd, CD33_151Eu, CD55_152Sm, CD366_153Eu, CD45RA_154Sm, CD152_156Gd, CD123_159Tb, CD69_160Dy, CD28_161Dy, Granzyme B_163Dy, CD127_165Ho, GPRC5D_166Er, CD19_167Er, CD269_168Er, CD25_169Tm, CD279_170Er, CD14_171Yb, CD38_172Yb, Vista_173Yb, HLA-DR_174Yb, CD56_176Yb) were combined.
2. It is critical for sample quality that the Smart Tubes after fixation are directly frozen at −80 °C in the supplied storage boxes and that no major temperature changes are applied afterwards.
3. The extracellular panel of antibodies comprises all antibodies except antibodies for active Caspase 3, CD152, and Granzyme-B. All the antibodies have been tested in a titration experiment to obtain the optimal concentration.

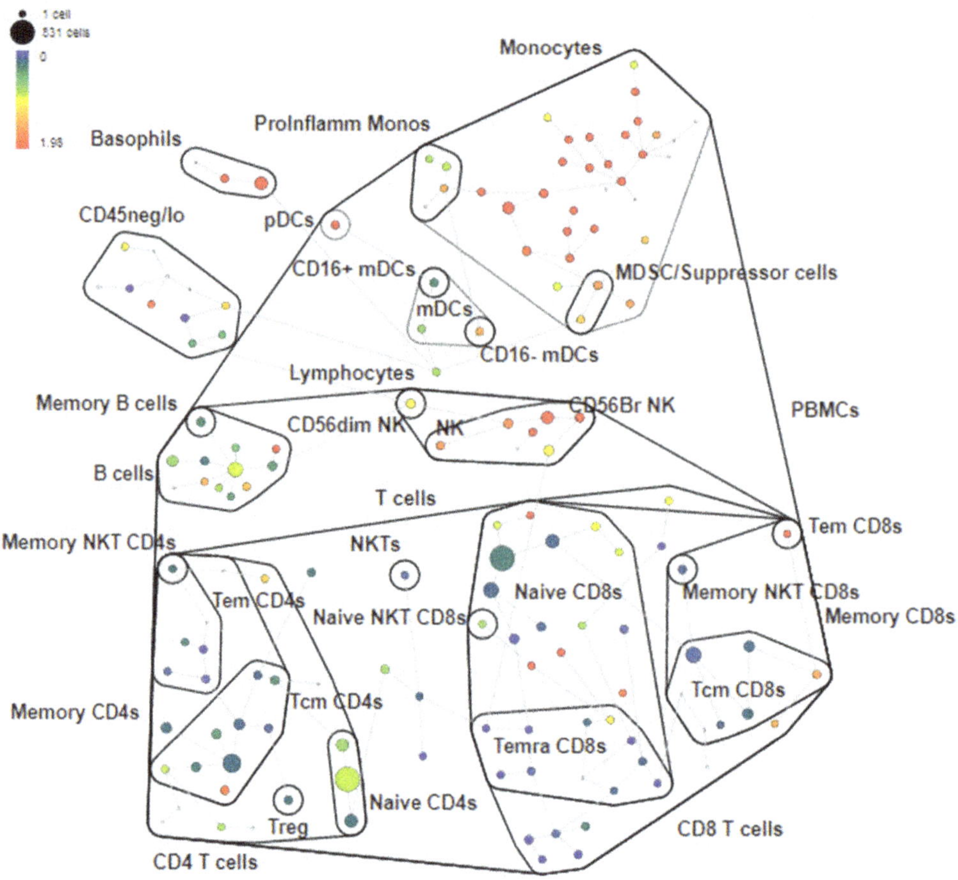

Fig. 1 SPADE tree of whole blood (*top*) and bone marrow (*bottom*) sample with cell populations annotated manually in Cytobank®. The node size represents the number of cells per node. The node colour represents the expression level of CD38. *SPADE*, spanning-tree progression analysis of density-normalized events; *NK*, natural killer; *ProInflamm Monos*, pro-inflammatory monocytes; *MDSC*, myeloid-derived suppressor cell; *PBMC*, peripheral blood mononuclear cell; *mDC*, myeloid dendritic cell; *pDC*, plasmacytoid dendritic cell; *NKT*, natural killer T cell; *Tcm*, central memory T cell; *Tem*, effector memory T cell; *Temra*, effector memory RA+ T cell; *Treg*, regulatory T cell

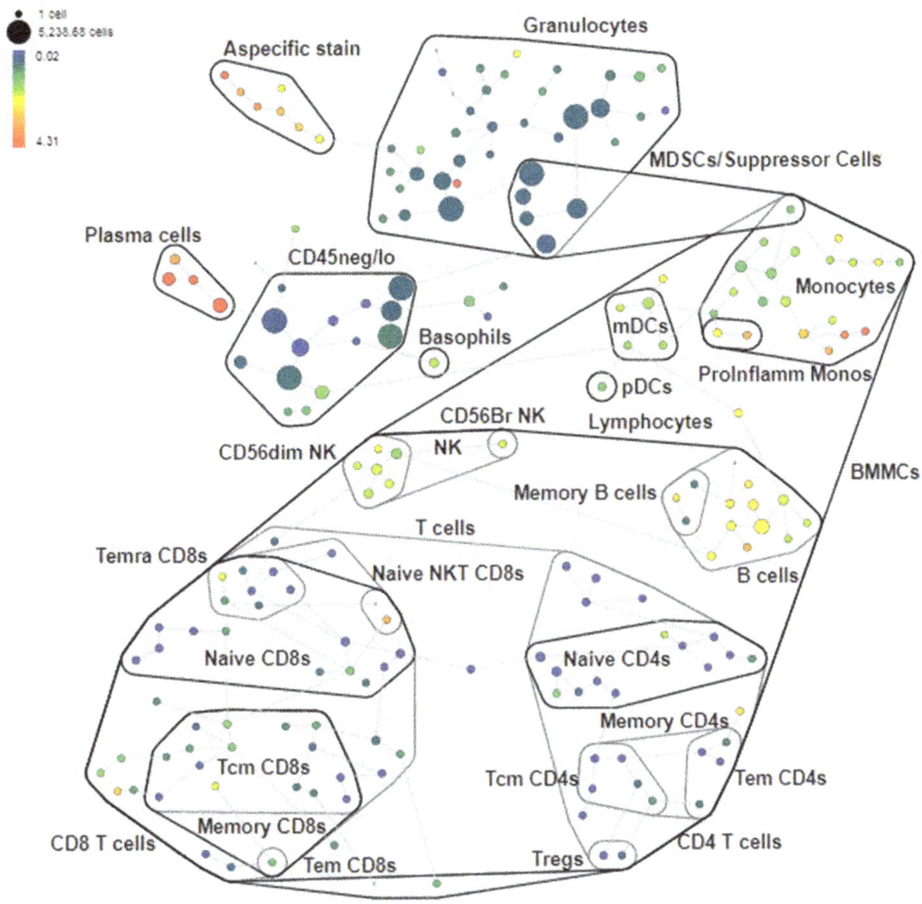

Fig. 1 (continued)

4. The intracellular panel consists of active Caspase 3, CD152, and Granzyme-B.
5. The Cell-ID™ 20-Plex Pd Barcoding Kit contains 20 unique combinations of six different Pd isotopes. This allows for barcoding of 20 samples at once. In our protocol barcoding of samples is done prior to acquisition on CyTOF. The samples can be combined and acquired on CyTOF as one multiplexed sample eliminating data collection variation. Samples can also be barcoded after thawing of the samples, allowing to combine samples after barcoding before staining, eliminating variations between staining of different samples. Performing the barcoding protocol at the start involves an extra permeabilization step and numerous centrifugation steps, resulting in a more limited yield of cells per sample. As we were interested in evaluation of rare cell populations, we decided to perform the barcoding after the staining procedure to optimize yield of cell numbers.

6. The concentration of Iridium needs to be titrated for individual cell types and experiments for optimal Cell-ID Intercalator staining. It is suggested not to exceed 1 μM intercalator concentration in the staining solution to avoid early failure of the detector.

Acknowledgments

The authors would like to thank Christoph Heuck for his suggestions and critical reading of the manuscript.

References

1. Bendall SC, Nolan GP, Roederer M, Chattopadhyay PK (2012) A deep profiler's guide to cytometry. Trends Immunol 33(7):323–332. https://doi.org/10.1016/j.it.2012.02.010
2. Spitzer MH, Nolan GP (2016) Mass Cytometry: single cells, many features. Cell 165(4):780–791. https://doi.org/10.1016/j.cell.2016.04.019
3. Lokhorst HM, Plesner T, Laubach JP, Nahi H, Gimsing P, Hansson M, Minnema MC, Lassen U, Krejcik J, Palumbo A, van de Donk NW, Ahmadi T, Khan I, Uhlar CM, Wang J, Sasser AK, Losic N, Lisby S, Basse L, Brun N, Richardson PG (2015) Targeting CD38 with daratumumab monotherapy in multiple myeloma. N Engl J Med 373(13):1207–1219. https://doi.org/10.1056/NEJMoa1506348
4. Lonial S, Weiss BM, Usmani SZ, Singhal S, Chari A, Bahlis NJ, Belch A, Krishnan A, Vescio RA, Mateos MV, Mazumder A, Orlowski RZ, Sutherland HJ, Blade J, Scott EC, Oriol A, Berdeja J, Gharibo M, Stevens DA, LeBlanc R, Sebag M, Callander N, Jakubowiak A, White D, de la Rubia J, Richardson PG, Lisby S, Feng H, Uhlar CM, Khan I, Ahmadi T, Voorhees PM (2016) Daratumumab monotherapy in patients with treatment-refractory multiple myeloma (SIRIUS): an open-label, randomised, phase 2 trial. Lancet 387(10027):1551–1560. https://doi.org/10.1016/S0140-6736(15)01120-4
5. Plesner T, Arkenau HT, Gimsing P, Krejcik J, Lemech C, Minnema MC, Lassen U, Laubach JP, Palumbo A, Lisby S, Basse L, Wang J, Sasser AK, Guckert ME, de Boer C, Khokhar NZ, Yeh H, Clemens PL, Ahmadi T, Lokhorst HM, Richardson PG (2016) Phase 1/2 study of daratumumab, lenalidomide, and dexamethasone for relapsed multiple myeloma. Blood 128(14):1821–1828. https://doi.org/10.1182/blood-2016-07-726729
6. Adams H, Stevenaert F, Krejcik J, Van der Borght K, Casneuf T, Smets T, Bald J, Abraham Y, Ceulemans H, Vanhoof G, Ahmadi T, Usmani SZ, Plesner T, Lonial S, van Kessel-Welmers B, Lokhorst HM, Mutis T, van de Donk NWCJ, Sasser AK (2016) High-parameter mass cytometry (CyTOF) evaluation of relapsed/refractory multiple myeloma (MM) Pts (Pts) treated with daratumumab supports immune modulation as a novel mechanism of action. Blood 128(22):4521
7. Qiu P, Simonds EF, Bendall SC, Gibbs KD Jr, Bruggner RV, Linderman MD, Sachs K, Nolan GP, Plevritis SK (2011) Extracting a cellular hierarchy from high-dimensional cytometry data with SPADE. Nat Biotechnol 29(10):886–891. https://doi.org/10.1038/nbt.1991

Chapter 5

Fluorescence In Situ Hybridization (FISH) in Multiple Myeloma

Erming Tian

Abstract

The application of fluorescence in situ hybridization (FISH) technology in diagnosis and molecular classification of cancer-risk has become an essential tool in the proceeding of personalized therapy. In multiple myeloma, the precise FISH detection of numerical and structural genetic aberrations can be carried out on metaphase chromosome spreads, interphase nuclei, and formalin fixed paraffin-embedded (FFPE) tissues. To dissect highly complex cancer genomes, a broad variety of novel DNA probes, which outpace supplies from commercial resources on the market, are also crucial to the advanced translational researches. Here, we provide the protocols for the creation of custom-made DNA probes and for conducting hybridizations on various targeting cells and tissues.

Key words Cancer cytogenetics, FISH, DNA probes

1 Introduction

As with other molecular genomic methods, e.g. Southern blotting and Northern blotting, the success of in situ hybridization depends on the stability of DNA double-strand, which can be repeatedly constituted through denaturing and annealing process. Under optimal conditions, DNA probes that are comprised of fluorochrome conjugated deoxynucleotide triphosphates complementarily affiliate to the counterpart DNA sequences to identify and quantify the targeted chromosomal segments. All abnormal genetic alterations including numerical amplification or deletion, structural rearrangements and translocations can be detected with the understanding that sopisticated DNA probes and FISH techniques are properly applied.

In multiple myeloma, the plasma cell dyscrasias arise due to aberrant genomic rearrangements during the lineage and terminal differentiation of B lymphocytes. The numerical aberrations in bone marrow and peripheral blood of patients diagnosed with the malignancy were initially observed by conventional karyotyping

Christoph Heuck and Niels Weinhold (eds.), *Multiple Myeloma: Methods and Protocols*, Methods in Molecular Biology, vol. 1792, https://doi.org/10.1007/978-1-4939-7865-6_5, © Springer Science+Business Media, LLC, part of Springer Nature 2018

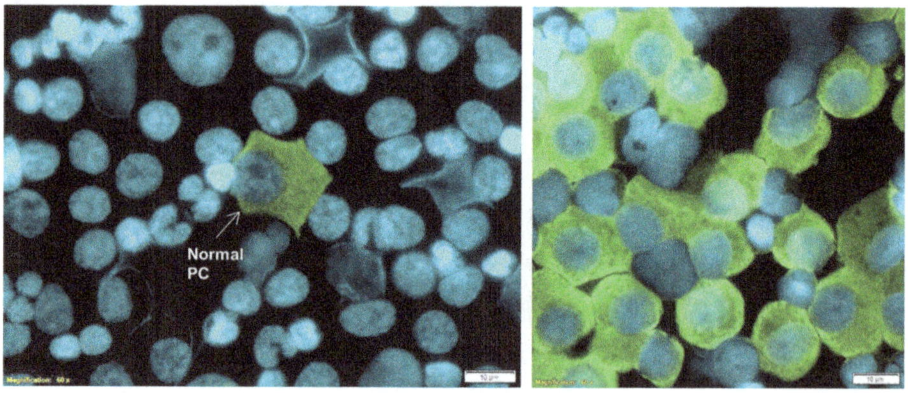

Fig. 1 Immunohistochemistry staining of the bone marrow aspirate from a patient with multiple myeloma with a Kappa-light chain (FITC-green, left) and a Lambda-light chain antibody (FITC-green, right) shows coexistence of normal plasma cell (Normal PC, left) that expresses Kappa-immunoglobulin (left) and myeloma cells (right) which express Lambda-immunoglobulin. The nuclei were stained with DAPI

with Giemsa stain (G-banding) [1–5]. Ever since, the molecular cytogenetic methodologies have provided evidence of much more complicated structural alterations. By combining karyotyping and FISH, chromosome breakpoints, translocation arrangements, and jumping/integration sites were discovered in myeloma genomes [6–16]. However, preparation of ideal metaphase chromosomes is highly restricted to the proliferative activity of cells under cell-culture condition (in vitro). In general, about 10% of myeloma cases can be successfully analyzed using G-banding method. For a large cohort of the patients, we developed a highly efficient interphase FISH (iFISH) technique to examine recurrent genetic lesions in intact cells [11]. Myeloma is a clonal disease which produces one type of light chain immunoglobulin (Kappa or Lambda) (Fig. 1). Precise detection of genetic aberrations in the tumor cells but not in normal plasma cells or in a range of heterogeneous cell populations in the bone marrow and blood is essential for the molecular diagnosis of the disease. Our iFISH approach of combining FISH and immunohistochemistry has succeeded to efficiently and accurately analyze the cytogenetics of thousands of samples from patients with myeloma (Fig. 2). Here, we provide the protocols for the creation of custom-made DNA probes and for conducting hybridizations on various target cells and tissues.

2 Materials

2.1 Creation of Custom-Made DNA Probes

1. Lennox L Broth base (LB) medium.
2. Bacterial incubator (37 °C).
3. Incubating shaker (37 °C, 225–250 rpm).

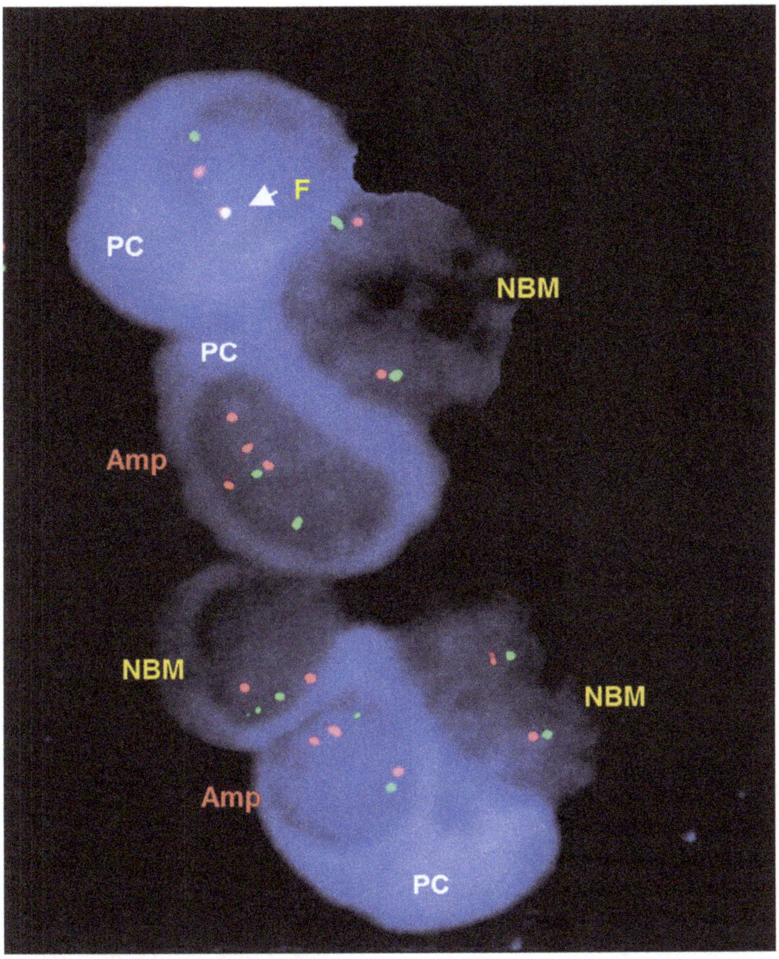

Fig. 2 Interphase FISH was applied to bone marrow cells from a patient with newly diagnosed multiple myeloma. Myeloma cells (PC) were defined by the stain of AMCA-conjugated anti-human Kappa light chain antibody (blue). The image illustrates normal signal pattern (2× green/2× red) in normal bone marrow cells (NBM), amplification (Amp) of the probe in red with extra copies of the signal in PC, and fusion of green and red probes turned in white (F)

4. Benchtop centrifuge with refrigeration.
5. Benchtop high speed microcentrifuge with refrigeration.
6. Chloramphenicol (34 mg per mL of 100% ethanol, store at −20 °C).
7. Kanamycin (10 mg per mL of milliQ water, store at −20 °C).
8. The NucleoBond PC20 kit (Takara-Clontech, CA) or other method if preferred.
9. Isopropanol (100%).
10. Glycerol (40% sterilized by autoclave).

11. Ethanol (70%).
12. Electrophoresis apparatus and power supply.
13. Agarose.
14. TAE buffer (50×).
15. Ethidium bromide or other DNA stains.
16. BamHI restriction endonuclease.
17. DNA ladder.
18. UV imaging system.
19. −80 °C freezer.
20. Nick Translation reaction kit (Abbott Molecular Inc. Des Plains, IL).
21. Fluorochrome green or red dUTP.
22. Human Cot-1 DNA or Human placental DNA.
23. Herring sperm DNA.
24. Sodium acetate (3 M, pH 5.0).
25. Bench-top cooler (−10 °C to room temperature) and water bath.
26. In situ hybridization buffer (*see* **Note 1**).

2.2 Slide Preparation for Interphase and Metaphase Fluorescence In Situ Hybridization

1. RPMI1640 medium.
2. Fetal bovine serum.
3. Histopaque-1077 or other density-filtration media (1.077 g/mL).
4. 1× Phosphate Buffered Saline (PBS).
5. Benchtop centrifuge.
6. Glass microscope slides (slide-labeler if preferred).
7. Shandon Cytospin centrifuge and accessories.
8. Hemacytometer.
9. Ethanol.
10. Coplin jars.
11. Dry oven.
12. Slide storage box.
13. −20 °C freezer.
14. Diamond pen.

2.3 Interphase Fluorescence In Situ Hybridization

1. 20× ultrapure SSC.
2. Molecular grade formamide (store at −20 °C in the dark).
3. milliQ water.
4. 70%, 85%, and 100% cold ethanol (store at −20 °C at least a day before use).

5. NaCl.
6. Na_2HPO_4.
7. NaH_2PO_4.
8. NP-40.
9. 10× PBS.
10. Rubber-Cement (*see* **Note 2**).
11. 90% formamide/2× SSC solution: mix deionized molecular grade formamide and 20× ultrapure SSC at ratio of 9:1 and adjust pH to 7.0 (*see* **Note 3**).
12. 2× SSC solution: at ratio of 1:9, mix 20× ultrapure SSC and milliQ water and adjust pH to 7.0 (*see* **Note 3**).
13. 50% formamide/2× SSC solution: at ratio of 5:1:4, mix 100% deionized molecular grade formamide, 20× ultrapure SSC, and milliQ and adjust pH to 7.0 (*see* **Note 3**).
14. 0.5 M $NaPO_4$ buffer—mix 0.5 M Na_2HPO_4 and 0.5 M NaH_2PO_4 and adjust pH to 7.5.
15. 1× PBD solution—add 10 mL NP-40 to 1000 mL 10× PBS solution, mix well. To make 1× PBD solution, dilute with water at ratio of 1:9 and adjust pH to 7 (*see* **Note 3**).
16. Antibody reaction buffer—dilute to final 50 mM $NaPO_4$ buffer and 0.15 M NaCl in milliQ water to pH 7.5, and store at 4 °C (*see* **Note 3**).
17. AMCA Goat-antibody to Human Kappa or Lambda light chain (Vector Laboratories, Burlingame, CA).
18. AMCA Rabbit-antibody to Goat IgH + L chains (Vector).
19. Antifade mounting solution.
20. Heating plate or oven (Hybrite).
21. Glass Coplin jar.
22. Digital pH meter.
23. Water bath.

2.4 Metaphase Fluorescence In Situ Hybridization

1. 20× ultrapure SSC.
2. Molecular grade Formamide (store at −20 °C in the dark).
3. milliQ water.
4. 0.01 M HCl solution.
5. Pepsin stock (10%) in water, store at −20 °C.
6. 1× PBS (pH 7.2).
7. Rubber-Cement (*see* **Note 2**).
8. Magnesium chloride hexahydrate to make 1 M $MgCl_2$ in water.
9. 1× PBS/0.05 M $MgCl_2$.

10. 1% formaldehyde: dilute 37% formaldehyde in 1× PBS/0.05 M $MgCl_2$ to final 1%.
11. 70%, 85%, and 100% ethanol (prepare with water and chill in a freezer (−20 °C) at least a day before use).
12. 50% formamide/2× SSC solution: at ratio of 5:1:4, mix 100% deionized molecular grade formamide, 20× ultrapure SSC, and milliQ and adjust pH to 7.0 (*see* **Note 3**).
13. 2× SSC solution: at ratio of 1:9, mix 20× ultrapure SSC and milliQ water and adjust pH to 7.0 (*see* **Note 3**).
14. 1× PBD solution—add 10 mL NP-40 to 1000 mL 10× PBS solution, mix well, dilute with water at ratio of 1:9 and adjust pH to 7 (*see* **Note 3**).
15. 0.01 M HCl/pepsin solution: 50 mL of 0.01 M HCl + 7 μL of 10% pepsin stock (*see* **Note 4**).
16. DAPI (4′,6-diamidino-2-phenylindole) (10 mg/mL).
17. Heating plate or oven (Hybrite).
18. Glass Coplin jar.
19. Digital pH meter.
20. Water bath.

2.5 Fluorescence In Situ Hybridization on Formalin Fixed Paraffin-Embedded Tissues

1. 20× ultrapure SSC.
2. Molecular grade formamide (store at −20 °C in the dark).
3. milliQ water.
4. 1× PBS (pH 7.2).
5. Xylene.
6. Ethanol.
7. milliQ water.
8. HCl.
9. Rubber-Cement (*see* **Note 2**).
10. Pepsin stock (10%) in water, store at −20 °C.
11. 8% sodium thiocyanate.
12. 70%, 85%, and 100% ethanol (prepare with water and chill in a freezer (−20 °C) at least a day before use).
13. 70% formamide/2× SSC: at ratio of 7:1:2, mix 100% deionized molecular grade formamide, 20× ultrapure SSC, and milliQ and adjust pH to 7.0 (*see* **Note 3**).
14. 50% formamide/2× SSC solution: at ratio of 5:1:4, mix 100% deionized molecular grade formamide, 20× ultrapure SSC, and milliQ and adjust pH to 7.0 (*see* **Note 3**).
15. 2× SSC solution: at ratio of 1:9, mix 20× ultrapure SSC and milliQ water and adjust pH to 7.0 (*see* **Note 3**).

16. 1× PBD solution—add 10 mL NP-40 to 1000 mL 10× PBS solution, mix well, dilute with water at ratio of 1:9 and adjust pH to 7 (*see* **Note 3**).
17. DAPI (4′,6-diamidino-2-phenylindole) (10 mg/mL).
18. 0.05% pepsin: at a ratio of 1:199, mix pepsin stock with 0.2 M HCl (*see* **Note 4**).
19. Heating plate or oven (Hybrite).
20. Glass Coplin jar.
21. Digital pH meter.
22. Water bath.

3 Methods

3.1 Creation of Custom-Made DNA Probes

1. The human bacterial artificial chromosome (BAC) library is a vast resource of large-insert genomic DNA clones that integrate the genetic landmarks into the draft sequence of the human genome [17]. The length and uniqueness of each BAC clone is ideal for making a customized DNA probe. The details of identifying a specific clone for the chromosomal segment of interest are available at the National Center for Biotechnology Information (NCBI, https://www.ncbi.nlm.nih.gov/genome/cyto/hbrc.shtml). As an example BAC clones for the human *BCL2* gene at chromosome 18q21 are shown in Fig. 3 (*see* **Note 5**).
2. Purchase the BAC clones through a vendor such as the BACPAC resources (CHORI, Oakland, CA) at https://bacpacresources.org.

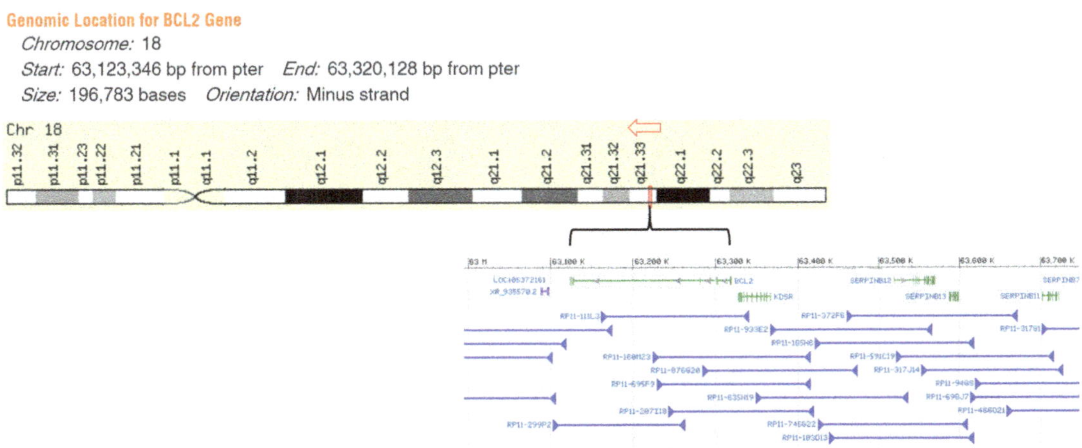

Fig. 3 The B-Cell CLL/Lymphoma 2 (*BCL2*) gene is located at 18q21.33. The full length genomic DNA of *BCL2* is ~197 kb. The NCBI database shows the alignment of BAC clones to *BCL2* locus and the adjacent regions. Accordingly, two clones of RP11-111J3 and RP11-299P2 combine the full genomic sequences of *BCL*. The probe for *BCL2* may be comprised of these BAC clones

3. Streak vial on a LB agar plate (containing 12.5 μg/mL chloramphenicol or 50 μg/mL of kanamycin as recommended by the vendor) to separate into individual colonies.
4. Inoculate a colony in 10 mL of LB with appropriate antibiotics. Incubate overnight at 37 °C and shaking at 250 rpm (*see* **Note 6**).
5. Aliquot 5 mL of LB and collect bacteria by centrifugation at 3000 rpm (1500–2000 × *g*) for 10 min and 4 °C
6. The NucleoBond PC20 kit provides all buffers and mini-columns. Follow the instruction to extract high purity BAC DNA (*see* **Note 7**).
7. From each mini-prep, digest 0.5–1 μg of BAC plasmids with the restriction endonuclease BamHI at 37 °C for >2 h.
8. Separate DNA bands by electrophoresis in 1% agarose gel and 1× TAE buffer, at 20–30 V overnight. The patterns of DNA bands indicate the identity of each clone (Fig. 4). The clones may be further verified using PCR or FISH.
9. Store the BAC clone by mixing bacteria/LB and 40% Glycerol at 1:1 ratio and keeping at −80 °C.
10. Use the following 50 μL reaction mixture to label BAC DNA (based on Nick Translation reaction kit from Abbott, *see* **Notes 8** and **9**):

27 μL	1 μg of BAC DNA
2.5 μL	0.2 mM of fluorochrome—green or red—conjugated dUTP
2.5 μL	0.1 mM of dTTP
3 μL	0.3 mM of dATP–dCTP–dGTP mix
5 μL	10× Nick translation buffer
10 μL	Nick translation enzymes

11. Incubate at 15 °C for 1–2 h (time needs to be adjusted regarding final DNA sizes) and 70 °C for 10 min.
12. Run 1/10 of Nick Translation products in 1.5% agarose gel and 1× TAE buffer, at 70–100 V for ≥1 h. Check DNA smear in each lane for the optimal reaction condition that fragments BAC DNA into a range of 300–1000 bp (Fig. 5).
13. To precipitate the DNA add the following to each reaction:

10 μL	Human Cot-1 DNA or placental DNA (1 μg/μL)
10 μL	Herring sperm DNA (1 μg/μL)
7 μL	3 M of sodium acetate, pH 5.0
200 μL	Cold 100% ethanol (−20 °C)

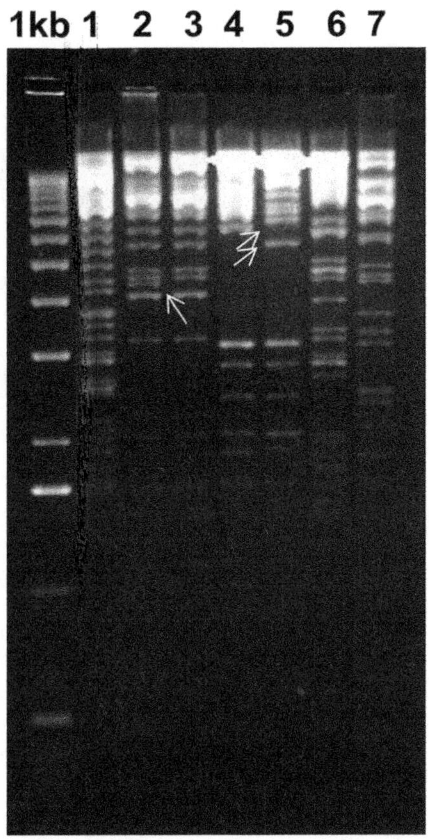

Fig. 4 DNA of seven BAC clones was purified using the mini-prep kit from Clontech. 1 μg of DNA was digested with the restriction endonuclease BamHI and separated in 1% TAE agarose gel. Lanes 2 and 3 are two BAC clones at the locus of a gene, and the electrophoresis shows the homologue sequences of two clones but differentiated by an extra band in lane 2 (arrow). Lane 4 and 5 show two BAC clones at another location but differentiated by extra bands (arrows). Lane 6 and 7 show different patterns of two BAC clones at the same gene locus. The gel demonstrates high quality of BAC DNA preparations with low background. 1 kb: 1 kb DNA ladder (Invitrogen)

14. Mix well and place at −20 °C for ≥30 min.
15. Collect DNA probes at maximum speed of benchtop centrifuge for 30 min, 4 °C.
16. Wash DNA pellet with 70% Ethanol once, collect the probe, and air-dry at room temperature.
17. Suspend DNA probes in 100 μL of in situ hybridization buffer.
18. Heat-denature at 75 °C for 10 min.
19. Block nonspecific genomic sequences at 37 °C for 30 min.
20. Store the probes at −20 °C and avoid direct light.

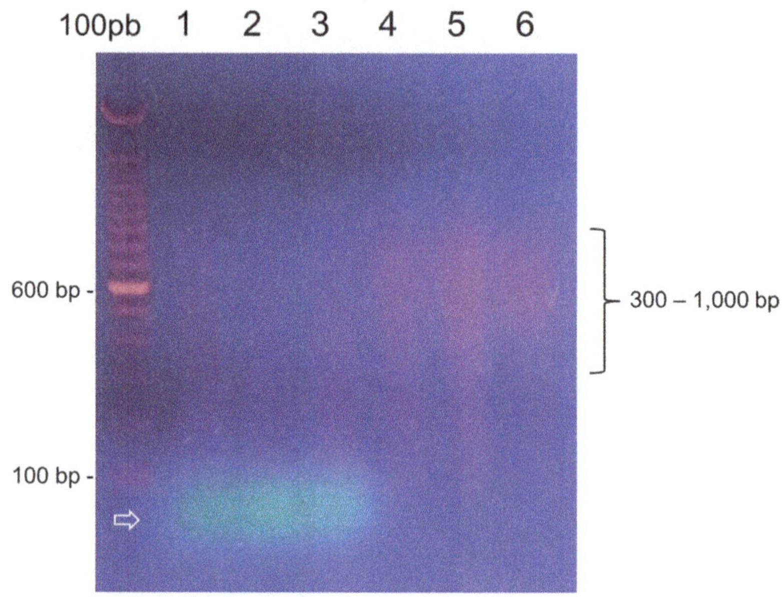

Fig. 5 Electrophoresis shows the sizes DNA of fragments after Nick Translation reactions. Lanes 1–3 are BAC DNA labeled with FITC-dUTP, lanes 4–6 are BAC DNA labeled with Spectrum-Red-dUTP. The ranges of the DNA smear (300–1000 bp) indicate the optimal reaction conditions. Free FITC-dUTP migrate the fastest (arrow). 100pb: 100 bp DNA ladder

3.2 Slide Preparation for Interphase and Metaphase Fluorescence In Situ Hybridization

1. Bone marrow aspirates and peripheral blood must be immediately mixed with anticoagulant Heparin or EDTA.
2. To remove erythrocytes, bone marrow or blood should be diluted in RPMI1640 + 5% fetal bovine serum at 1:1 or 1:5 ratio. Gently lay diluted cells onto Histopaque-1077 medium (density = 1.077).
3. Centrifuge cells at speed of 600–800 × *g* (or 1800–2000 rpm) for 25 min at room temperature without break.
4. Carefully harvest the layer of leukocytes at the interface.
5. Wash leukocytes at least once with RPMI1640 medium.
6. Use a hemacytometer to get cell counts and adjust to 10^6/mL.
7. If using a Shandon Cytospin centrifuge, assemble a Cytoclip, a glass slide, a paper filter card, and a sample chamber together and add 0.1 mL of cell suspension in the chamber. Centrifuge for 5 min at 1000 rpm, at room temperature (*see* **Note 10**).
8. After first spot was done, dissemble the clip and turn slide around 180° and add 0.1 mL cell suspension in the chamber. Centrifuge for 5 min at 1000 rpm to attach cells on the second spot of the same slide (*see* **Note 11**).

9. After Cytospin, immediately dissemble the clips and fully submerge slides in a Coplin jar filled with 100% Ethanol to fix cells for 5–10 min at room temperature (*see* **Note 12**).
10. Mark cell spots with a diamond pen on back of slides.
11. Bake fixed slides at 37 °C in a dry oven overnight.
12. Slides can be stored at −20 °C (*see* **Note 13**).

3.3 Interphase Fluorescence In Situ Hybridization

1. Take the slides from −20 °C and immediately submerge into prewarmed 90% formamide/2× SSC solution at 37 °C for 8 min.
2. Quench slides in cold (−20 °C) 70% Ethanol for 3 min, cold 85% Ethanol for 3 min, and then cold 100% Ethanol for 3 min. Air dry the slides in upright position on paper towels.
3. Add 10 μL of 1:1 mixed fluorochrome red and green probes to each spot.
4. Gently cover each spot with a thin circle coverslip (do not press on coverslip), and then apply Rubber-Cement glue around the coverslips and dry the glue at room temperature in vented hood.
5. Incubate the slides in the Hybrite thermal plate at 75 °C for 15 min (denature) and 42 °C for 20 h (hybridization).
6. Peel off Rubber-Cement seal and remove coverslip.
7. Submerge slides in prewarmed 50% formamide/2× SSC solution pH7.0 at 50–55 °C for 30 min (*see* **Note 14**).
8. Transfer slides to prewarmed 2× SSC solution pH7.0 at 37 °C for 8 min.
9. Wash slides in 1× PBD for 3 min at room temperature.
10. For the light chain (Kappa or Lambda) antibody staining dilute AMCA Goat-antibody to Human Kappa or Lambda light chain at 1:20 ratio in the dilution buffer and add 100 μL to each spot. Stain for 30 min at room temperature.
11. Wash in 1× PBD twice (5 min/wash).
12. Dilute AMCA Rabbit-antibody to Goat IgH + L chains at 1:40 ratio in the dilution buffer and add 100 μL to each spot. Stain for 30 min at room temperature.
13. Wash in 1× PBD twice (5 min/wash).
14. Drain the solution but don't let completely dry. Add 10 μL of Antifade mounting solution to each spot and cover with a rectangle coverslip (20 × 60 cm).
15. Store slides at 4 °C.

3.4 Metaphase Fluorescence In Situ Hybridization

1. Scan fixed slides using phase microscopy for an area of higher mitotic index and good metaphase spreads.
2. Select an area of the slide to be hybridized and mark the back of the slide with a diamond pen.
3. Immerse slide in prewarmed 0.01 M HCl/pepsin solution for 4 min 30 s at 37 °C.
4. Wash in 1× PBS twice for 5 min at room temperature.
5. Immerse slide in PBS/$MgCl_2$ solution for 5 min.
6. Incubate in 1% formaldehyde solution for 10 min at room temperature.
7. Wash in 1× PBS for 5 min with gentle intermittent agitation.
8. Submerge slide in cold (−20 °C) 70% ethanol for 3 min, cold 80% ethanol for 3 min, and cold 100% ethanol for 3 min.
9. Air dry slides.
10. Add 10 μL of 1:1 mixed fluorochrome red and green probes to each spot.
11. Gently cover each spot with a thin circle coverslip (do not press on coverslip), and then apply Rubber-Cement around the coverslips and dry the glue at room temperature in vented hood.
12. Incubate the slides in the Hybrite thermal plate at 75 °C for 15 min (denature) and 37–42 °C for 20 h (hybridization).
13. Peel off Rubber-Cement seal and remove coverslip.
14. Submerge slides in 50% formamide/2× SSC solution pH7.0 (50–55 °C) for 30 min.
15. Transfer slides to 2× SSC solution pH7.0 (37 °C) for 8 min.
16. Wash in 1× PBD for 3 min at room temperature.
17. Dilute DAPI stock (10 mg/mL) into 50 mL of 1× PBS at 1:10,000 ratio in a Coplin jar, and stain slide for 5–10 min.
18. Wash in 1× PBD for 3 min at room temperature.
19. Drain the solution but do not let completely dry. Add 10 μL of Antifade mounting solution to each spot and cover with a rectangle coverslip (20 × 60 mm).
20. Store slides at 4 °C.

3.5 Fluorescence In Situ Hybridization on Formalin Fixed Paraffin-Embedded Tissues (See Note 15)

1. Heat slides at 60 °C in an oven (Hybrite) for at least 2 h until the paraffin is completely liquidized.
2. Immerse heated slides immediately in Xylene at 55 °C for 5 min, repeat twice in fresh Xylene at 55 °C.
3. Rehydrate slides in 100%–90%–70% ethanol series at room temperature for 3 min each.
4. Wash in milliQ water for 3 min.

5. Pretreat slides with 0.2 M HCl for 20 min at room temperature.
6. Wash in milliQ water for 3 min.
7. Incubate slides in prewarmed 8% sodium thiocyanate in milliQ water for 30 min at 80 °C.
8. Wash in milliQ water for 3 min.
9. Treat slides in prewarmed 0.05% pepsin at 37 °C for 24 min.
10. Wash in milliQ for 3 min.
11. Wash in 1× PBS pH 7.0 for 5 min at room temperature.
12. Wash in 2× SSC pH 7.0 for 5 min at room temperature.
13. Incubate slides in preheated 72 °C 70% formamide/2× SSC for 15 min.
14. Immediately submerge slides in cold (−20 °C) 70%, 85% and 100% Ethanol for 3 min each.
15. Air dry slides till traceless.
16. Add 10 μL of 1:1 mixed fluorochrome red and green probes to each spot.
17. Gently cover each spot with a thin circle coverslip (do not press on coverslip), and then apply Rubber-Cement around the coverslips and dry the glue at room temperature in vented hood.
18. Incubate the slides in the Hybrite thermal plate at 75 °C for 15 min (denature) and 37–42 °C for 20 h (hybridization).
19. Peel off Rubber-Cement seal and remove coverslip.
20. Submerge slides in 50% formamide/2× SSC pH7.0 solution (50–55 °C) for 30 min.
21. Transfer slides to 2× SSC solution pH7.0 (37 °C) for 8 min.
22. Wash in 1× PBD for 3 min at room temperature.
23. Dilute DAPI stock (10 mg/mL) into 50 mL of 1× PBS at 1:10,000 ratio in a Coplin jar, and stain slide for 5–10 min.
24. Wash in 1× PBD for 3 min at room temperature.
25. Drain the solution but do not let completely dry. Add 10 μL of Antifade mounting solution to each spot and cover with a rectangle coverslip (20 × 60 cm).
26. Store slides at 4 °C.

4 Notes

1. We use the DakoCytomation "DNA In Situ Hybridization Solution" but hybridization buffers sold by other venders may also work.

2. Elmer's brand Rubber-Cement has the solvent that does not affect DNA hybridization. We have tried other brands but did not get convincing results.
3. Control of pH is critical: use a digital pH meter, but not pH paper strips.
4. Add pepsin stock in a Coplin jar before HCl.
5. The ideal size of a BAC insert should cover full length of the gene; otherwise, several BAC clones may be selected.
6. Several colonies need to be selected and examined for the insert.
7. The purity of the BAC plasmid is crucial to the quality of probes for FISH.
8. All steps should be carried out without bright light
9. The biomolecules such as biotin and digoxigenin conjugated dUTP may substitute fluorochrome directly labeled deoxynucleotide triphosphates in Nick Translation reactions. The incorporated biomolecules are amplified using avidin or antibodies conjugated with fluorochrome-dyes. The secondary development may generate brighter signals of the probes and also increase background.
10. Briefly vortex the tube and make sure of loading the cells but not the supernatant to the funnels.
11. Do not use double-channel sample chamber to make two spots at the same time. This kind of products not only leak but also fail to distribute cells evenly.
12. Overnight fixation is unnecessary but doesn't affect FISH.
13. Avoid repeatedly freeze and thaw of fixed slides.
14. Incubation temperature depends on the stability of DNA double strand between the probe and targeted chromosome.
15. Only tissues fixed in formalin or paraformaldehyde and paraffin-embedded can be used in this protocol. The thickness of tissue section should be at 3–5 micron.

References

1. Das KC, Aikat BK (1967) Chromosomal abnormalities in multiple myeloma. Blood 30(6):738–748
2. Philip P, Drivsholm A (1976) G-banding analysis of complex aneuploidy in multiple myeloma bone marrow cells. Blood 47(1):69–77
3. Liang W, Hopper JE, Rowley JD (1979) Karyotypic abnormalities and clinical aspects of patients with multiple myeloma and related paraproteinemic disorders. Cancer 44(2): 630–644
4. Dewald GW, Kyle RA, Hicks GA, Greipp PR (1985) The clinical significance of cytogenetic studies in 100 patients with multiple myeloma, plasma cell leukemia, or amyloidosis. Blood 66(2):380–390
5. Gould J, Alexanian R, Goodacre A, Pathak S, Hecht B, Barlogie B (1988) Plasma cell karyotype in multiple myeloma. Blood 71(2): 453–456
6. Flactif M, Zandecki M, Lai JL, Bernardi F, Obein V, Bauters F, Facon T (1995) Interphase

fluorescence in situ hybridization (FISH) as a powerful tool for the detection of aneuploidy in multiple myeloma. Leukemia 9(12):2109–2114

7. Lai JL, Zandecki M, Mary JY, Bernardi F, Izydorczyk V, Flactif M, Morel P, Jouet JP, Bauters F, Facon T (1995) Improved cytogenetics in multiple myeloma: a study of 151 patients including 117 patients at diagnosis. Blood 85(9):2490–2497
8. Calasanz MJ, Cigudosa JC, Odero MD, Ferreira C, Ardanaz MT, Fraile A, Carrasco JL, Sole F, Cuesta B, Gullon A (1997) Cytogenetic analysis of 280 patients with multiple myeloma and related disorders: primary breakpoints and clinical correlations. Genes Chromosomes Cancer 18(2):84–93
9. Chesi M, Nardini E, Brents LA, Schrock E, Ried T, Kuehl WM, Bergsagel PL (1997) Frequent translocation t(4;14)(p16.3;q32.3) in multiple myeloma is associated with increased expression and activating mutations of fibroblast growth factor receptor 3. Nat Genet 16(3):260–264. https://doi.org/10.1038/ng0797-260
10. Feinman R, Sawyer J, Hardin J, Tricot G (1997) Cytogenetics and molecular genetics in multiple myeloma. Hematol Oncol Clin North Am 11(1):1–25
11. Shaughnessy J, Tian E, Sawyer J, Bumm K, Landes R, Badros A, Morris C, Tricot G, Epstein J, Barlogie B (2000) High incidence of chromosome 13 deletion in multiple myeloma detected by multiprobe interphase FISH. Blood 96(4):1505–1511
12. Keung YK, Yung C, Wong JW, Shah F, Cobos E, Tonk V (1998) Unusual presentation of multiple myeloma with "jumping translocation" involving 1q21. A case report and review of the literature. Cancer Genet Cytogenet 106(2):135–139
13. Sawyer JR, Tricot G, Mattox S, Jagannath S, Barlogie B (1998) Jumping translocations of chromosome 1q in multiple myeloma: evidence for a mechanism involving decondensation of pericentromeric heterochromatin. Blood 91(5):1732–1741
14. Sawyer JR, Tricot G, Lukacs JL, Binz RL, Tian E, Barlogie B, Shaughnessy J Jr (2005) Genomic instability in multiple myeloma: evidence for jumping segmental duplications of chromosome arm 1q. Genes Chromosomes Cancer 42(1):95–106. https://doi.org/10.1002/gcc.20109
15. Hanamura I, Stewart JP, Huang Y, Zhan F, Santra M, Sawyer JR, Hollmig K, Zangarri M, Pineda-Roman M, van Rhee F, Cavallo F, Burington B, Crowley J, Tricot G, Barlogie B, Shaughnessy JD Jr (2006) Frequent gain of chromosome band 1q21 in plasma-cell dyscrasias detected by fluorescence in situ hybridization: incidence increases from MGUS to relapsed myeloma and is related to prognosis and disease progression following tandem stem-cell transplantation. Blood 108(5):1724–1732. https://doi.org/10.1182/blood-2006-03-009910
16. Tian E, Sawyer JR, Heuck CJ, Zhang Q, van Rhee F, Barlogie B, Epstein J (2014) In multiple myeloma, 14q32 translocations are nonrandom chromosomal fusions driving high expression levels of the respective partner genes. Genes Chromosomes Cancer 53(7):549–557. https://doi.org/10.1002/gcc.22165
17. Osoegawa K, Mammoser AG, Wu C, Frengen E, Zeng C, Catanese JJ, de Jong PJ (2001) A bacterial artificial chromosome library for sequencing the complete human genome. Genome Res 11(3):483–496. https://doi.org/10.1101/gr.169601

Chapter 6

Whole Exome Sequencing in Multiple Myeloma to Identify Somatic Single Nucleotide Variants and Key Translocations Involving Immunoglobulin Loci and *MYC*

Brian A. Walker

Abstract

Multiple myeloma is a malignancy of terminally differentiated plasma cells in the bone marrow. These plasma cells produce high levels of immunoglobulin which cause end-organ damage. Rearrangements within the immunoglobulin loci are a physiological part of B cell development, but these DNA level double-strand breaks may result in interchromosomal translocations. There are five main translocations involving the Ig loci: t(4;14) 12%, t(6;14) 1%, t(11;14) 15%, t(14;16) 3%, and t(14;20) 2%. These are primary events, found in all cells within the tumor clone and are associated with different prognosis. The t(4;14), t(14;16), and t(14;20) are associated with a poor prognosis, whereas the others are associated with a more favorable prognosis. Rearrangements at the *MYC* locus are also associated with a poor prognosis and increased expression of *MYC*. *MYC* rearrangements are frequent (25%) and involve interchromosomal translocations involving Ig loci or other partners, but also include intrachromosomal inversions, duplications and deletions. As such, the Ig and MYC loci are key players in the myeloma genome and including these in any genomic studies is key to understanding the relationship with other abnormalities. We have designed a custom capture of the Ig and *MYC* loci which can be added to exome or targeted captures to inform on these key events. This saves on performing additional tests to determine these events, which are generally mandatory for any genetic investigations in myeloma. This custom capture is also relevant to other B cell malignancies where MYC and Ig translocations occur.

Key words Multiple myeloma, Whole exome sequencing, Translocations, Immunoglobulin, MYC, Rearrangements, Somatic mutations

1 Introduction

Multiple myeloma (MM) is a malignancy of terminally differentiated plasma cells [1]. The genetic abnormalities underlying disease initiation and progression have been studied using a variety of techniques from fluorescence in situ hybridization (FISH), gene expression profiling, mapping arrays, and more recently genome sequencing studies [2–9]. Most sequencing studies are currently concentrated on whole exome sequencing (WES) in the research field to identify recurrently mutated genes in primary patient

Christoph Heuck and Niels Weinhold (eds.), *Multiple Myeloma: Methods and Protocols*, Methods in Molecular Biology, vol. 1792, https://doi.org/10.1007/978-1-4939-7865-6_6, © Springer Science+Business Media, LLC, part of Springer Nature 2018

samples [7, 9–12]. In addition, the information can be used to generate copy number data, infer subclonal populations and identify driver abnormalities leading to clonal outgrowth, resistance to treatment, and disease progression [7, 13–15].

The most frequent mutations in MM have been identified as *KRAS* (21%), *NRAS* (19%), *DIS3* (10%), *BRAF* (8%), *FAM46C* (5%), *TRAF3* (4%), and *TP53* (3.5%) [7, 9, 11]. In addition, copy number changes at 1p32.3 (*CDKN2C*), 1p12 (*FAM46C*), 1q21 (*CKS1B*), and 17p13.1 (*TP53*) are key prognostic indicators [8, 16, 17]. WES is capable of identifying these key abnormalities, which can be integrated with other somatic mutations present to determine clonal dynamics in the tumor population. However, these events are considered secondary to the initiating events in MM which are translocations involving the immunoglobulin (Ig) loci or hyperdiploidy involving trisomies of chromosomes 5, 9, 15, and 19 [1]. While WES is capable of identifying hyperdiploid samples it is not able to detect rearrangements involving the Ig loci, as these regions are not included in standard exome captures.

The translocations of interest mainly involve the *IGH* heavy chain locus on chromosome 14, but may also involve the light chain loci, *IGK* and *IGL*, on chromosomes 2 and 22 [18–20]. These are complex loci that in B cells undergo rearrangements at the DNA level in order to generate functional and diverse antibody molecules [21]. This is a multi-step process by which diversity (D) and joining (J) segments rearrange by means of recombination activating gene 1 (RAG1) and RAG2, which mediate DNA cleavage. Subsequently variable (V) segments rearrange with the D-J segment to create a functional V(D)J rearrangement with an IgM isotype. These events happen early on in B cell development during the pre- and pro-B cell stage. During maturation, and in response to a secondary infection, the Ig loci undergoes class switch recombination, mediated by activation induced cytidine deaminase (AID). In this process switch regions 5′ of the constant regions recombine to place the V(D)J rearrangement upstream of a different constant region, resulting in a change in isotype, for example to IgG1.

In MM, translocations occur predominantly during class switch recombination but can also occur during V(D)J rearrangements [22]. The main translocations detected in MM are the t(4;14) (12%), t(11;14) (15%), t(14;16) (3%), t(14;20) (2%), and the t(6;14) (1%). These can be divided in those associated with a poor prognosis (t(4;14), t(14;16) and t(14;20)) and those associated with a neutral prognosis (t(11;14) and t(6;14)) [2]. Although the *IGH* locus is the most common partner, rearrangements involving the light chain loci produce the same downstream effects. Given the association with patient outcome, it is important to stratify patients according to these translocation groups in downstream analyses.

Rearrangements involving the *MYC* loci at 8q24 are also common in MM (25%) and are associated with a poor prognosis [14, 23, 24]. The rearrangements at 8q24 may also involve the Ig loci but only in up to 35% of rearrangements. The other 65% of *MYC* rearrangements involve diverse loci across the genome, but are associated with recruitment of superenhancers to *MYC*, leading to overexpression of the gene. Common non-Ig partners include *FAM46C* (1p12), *FOXO3* (6q21), and *TXNDC5* (6q24.3), all of which have active superenhancers in MM cells. The breakpoints on 8q24 are not localized to a particular region and can occur 5′ or 3′ of *MYC* and up to 1.5 Mb away from the gene. Again, standard WES cannot identify these key translocations in MM.

In order to identify the key translocations in MM at the same time as performing WES we have designed a capture region encompassing the V segments of the *IGH/IGK* and *IGL* loci as well as the entire D-J and constant regions. In addition, we have included 2 Mb surrounding the *MYC* locus to identify these critical rearrangements. This capture region adds approximately 4.2 Mb of sequencing to a WES capture but can also be added on to targeted panels for clinical utility in a diagnostic setting. Using the additional capture region negates the need for extra testing for translocations in MM by FISH or gene expression profiling. The capture region is also applicable to other B cell malignancies where Ig translocations or *MYC* rearrangements are important, including diffuse large B cell lymphoma, mantle cell lymphoma, follicular lymphoma, and Burkitt's lymphoma.

2 Materials

2.1 Equipment

Lab areas should be divided into pre- and post-PCR to prevent contamination of amplified products into the original DNA sample.

2.2 Pre-PCR Area

1. Ice machine.
2. Ethanol (100% v/v).
3. 1N NaOH.
4. Nuclease-free water.
5. Pipettes, various volumes (0.5–1000 μL).
6. Filter tips, various volumes (0.1–1000 μL).
7. 96-well PCR plates.
8. Microplate centrifuge.
9. Magnetic stand-16.
10. PCR machine.
11. Vortexer.

12. Eppendorf Speed-Vac.
13. Heat block for 1.5 mL centrifuge tubes.
14. 50 mL Falcon tubes.
15. 15 mL Falcon tubes.
16. RNase/DNase-free water.
17. Lo-bind 1.5 mL RNase/DNase-free tubes.
18. 0.2 mL RNase/DNase-free 8-strip tubes and caps.
19. 48-well PCR plates.
20. Reagent reservoirs.
21. EB (elution buffer; 10 mM Tris–HCl, pH 8.5).
22. DNA clean and concentrator-5 kit.
23. Qubit fluorometer and double-stranded DNA quantification reagents.
24. KAPA Hyper Plus Kit (stored at −20 °C):
    (a) 5× Fragmentation Enzyme.
    (b) 10× Fragmentation Buffer.
    (c) Fragmentation Conditioning Solution.
    (d) End Repair & A-tailing Buffer.
    (e) End Repair & A-tailing Enzyme Mix.
    (f) Ligation Buffer, 900 μL.
    (g) DNA Ligase.
    (h) KAPA HiFi HotStart ReadyMix 2×, 690 μL.
25. Nimblegen SeqCap EZ Adapter Kit A (stored at −20 °C):
    (a) Pre-LM-PCR Oligos 1 & 2.
    (b) Water, PCR Grade.
    (c) SeqCap EZ Adapter A2 (A002 CGATGT).
    (d) SeqCap EZ Adapter A4 (A004 TGACCA).
    (e) SeqCap EZ Adapter A5 (A005 ACAGTG).
    (f) SeqCap EZ Adapter A6 (A006 GCCAAT).
    (g) SeqCap EZ Adapter A7 (A007 CAGATC).
    (h) SeqCap EZ Adapter A12 (A0012 CTTGTA).
    (i) SeqCap EZ Adapter A13 (A0013 AGTCAA).
    (j) SeqCap EZ Adapter A14 (A0014 AGTTCC).
    (k) SeqCap EZ Adapter A15 (A0015 ATGTCA).
    (l) SeqCap EZ Adapter A16 (A0016 CCGTCC).
    (m) SeqCap EZ Adapter A18 (A0018 GTCCGC).
    (n) SeqCap EZ Adapter A19 (A0019 GTGAAA).

26. Nimblegen SeqCap EZ Adapter Kit B (stored at −20 °C):
    (a) Pre-LM-PCR Oligos 1 & 2.
    (b) Water, PCR Grade.
    (c) SeqCap EZ Adapter A1 (A001 ATCACG).
    (d) SeqCap EZ Adapter A3 (A003 TTAGGC).
    (e) SeqCap EZ Adapter A8 (A008 ACTTGA).
    (f) SeqCap EZ Adapter A9 (A009 GATCAG).
    (g) SeqCap EZ Adapter A10 (A010 TAGCTT).
    (h) SeqCap EZ Adapter A11 (A011 GGCTAC).
    (i) SeqCap EZ Adapter A20 (A020 GTGGCC).
    (j) SeqCap EZ Adapter A21 (A021 GTTTCG).
    (k) SeqCap EZ Adapter A22 (A022 CGTACG).
    (l) SeqCap EZ Adapter A23 (A023 GAGTGG).
    (m) SeqCap EZ Adapter A25 (A025 ACTGAT).
    (n) SeqCap EZ Adapter A27 (A027 ATTCCT).
27. Nimblegen SeqCap HE-Oligo Kit A (stored at −20 °C):
    (a) SeqCap HE Universal Oligo.
    (b) Water, PCR Grade.
    (c) SeqCap HE Oligo Index 2.
    (d) SeqCap HE Oligo Index 4.
    (e) SeqCap HE Oligo Index 5.
    (f) SeqCap HE Oligo Index 6.
    (g) SeqCap HE Oligo Index 7.
    (h) SeqCap HE Oligo Index 12.
    (i) SeqCap HE Oligo Index 13.
    (j) SeqCap HE Oligo Index 14.
    (k) SeqCap HE Oligo Index 15.
    (l) SeqCap HE Oligo Index 16.
    (m) SeqCap HE Oligo Index 18.
    (n) SeqCap HE Oligo Index 19.
28. Nimblegen SeqCap HE-Oligo Kit B (stored at −20 °C):
    (a) SeqCap HE Universal Oligo.
    (b) Water, PCR Grade.
    (c) SeqCap HE Oligo Index 1.
    (d) SeqCap HE Oligo Index 3.
    (e) SeqCap HE Oligo Index 8.
    (f) SeqCap HE Oligo Index 9.

   (g) SeqCap HE Oligo Index 10.
   (h) SeqCap HE Oligo Index 11.
   (i) SeqCap HE Oligo Index 20.
   (j) SeqCap HE Oligo Index 21.
   (k) SeqCap HE Oligo Index 22.
   (l) SeqCap HE Oligo Index 23.
   (m) SeqCap HE Oligo Index 25.
   (n) SeqCap HE Oligo Index 27.

29. Nimblegen SeqCap EZ Pure Capture Bead Kit (stored at 2–8 °C):
   (a) SeqCap Capture Beads, 10 mL.
   (b) SeqCap Purification Beads, 30 mL.

30. Nimblegen SeqCap EZ Accessory Kit v.2 (stored at −20 °C):
   (a) KAPA HiFi HotStart ReadyMix, 2 × 1.25 mL.
   (b) Post-LM-PCR Oligos 1 & 2.
   (c) COT-1 Human DNA.
   (d) Water, DNA Grade.

31. Nimblegen Capture Custom Oligos (stored at −20 °C):
   (a) Nimblegen/Roche IRN: 4000024560. This contains the coordinates for the Ig and *MYC* loci, which can be added as custom content to any exome or targeted panel design. These additional baits allow identification of translocations into the Ig loci (H/κ/λ) and rearrangements within 2 Mb of *MYC*.

32. Nimblegen SeqCap EZ Hybridization and Wash Kit (stored at −20 °C):
   (a) 2× Hybridization Buffer.
   (b) Hybridization Component A.
   (c) 2.5× Bead Wash Buffer.
   (d) 10× Wash Buffer I.
   (e) 10× Wash Buffer II.
   (f) 10× Wash Buffer III.
   (g) 10× Stringent Buffer.

33. KAPA Illumina Library Quantitation Kit (stored at −20 °C):
   (a) KAPA SYBR® FAST qPCR Master Mix 2×, 5 mL.
   (b) Primer Premix 10×.
   (c) KAPA SYBR® FAST ROX Low 50×, 200 μL.
   (d) KAPA SYBR® FAST ROX High 50×, 200 μL.
   (e) DNA Standards 1–6.

34. AmpureXP Beads (stored at 2–8 °C).

2.3 Post-PCR Area

1. Thermal Cycler.
2. Quantitative Real-time PCR machine.
3. Pipettes, various volumes (0.5–1000 μL).
4. Filter tips, various volumes (0.1–1000 μL).
5. Magnetic stand-6 for 1.5 mL tubes.
6. Vortexer.
7. Agilent TapeStation.
8. Agilent TapeStation reagents (stored at 2–8 °C).
9. 50 mL Falcon tubes.
10. 15 mL Falcon tubes.
11. Lo-bind 1.5 mL RNase/DNase-free tubes.
12. RNase/DNase-free water.
13. 10% Tween 20 solution.
14. HPLC water.
15. EB (elution buffer; 10 mM Tris–Cl, pH 8.5).

3 Methods

3.1 Preparation of DNA

1. A maximum of 48 samples may be processed together in a plate format, which consists of 24 tumor/non-tumor pairs. Tumor DNA should be from CD138 selected cells originating from MM bone marrow aspirates, extramedullary biopsies or peripheral blood (plasma cell leukemia). Non-tumor DNA from the same patient should be used as a control sample in order to determine true somatic variants. For MM patients DNA from the buffy coat of a peripheral blood sample can be used. However, in a PCL patient the circulating tumor cells mean this cannot be used as a control. In this case the blood sample may be sequentially selected for tumor cells (using CD138 sorting) and T cells (using CD3 sorting) to obtain a suitable matched control sample.
2. *Optional*: Genomic TapeStation can be run on all samples to determine that the DNA is high molecular weight and free from degradation.
3. DNA should be eluted in a buffer free of EDTA, such as EB. EDTA will inhibit the enzymatic fragmentation step. DNA eluted in buffers containing EDTA should be cleaned up using ethanol precipitation or column-based methods, e.g., DNA Clean & Concentrator (*see* **Note 1**).
4. DNA must be quantitated using a method that measures only DNA, not contaminating RNA or free nucleotides, such as the HS Qubit reagents. If the concentration is above 50 ng/μL repeat the quantification with the BR Qubit reagents to obtain

an accurate measurement. Before proceeding further the DNA concentration should be ≥6.66 ng/μL. If the concentration is <6.66 ng/μL, but the total amount of DNA is >100 ng, the sample should be concentrated (*see* **Notes 2 and 3**).

3.2 DNA Dilution and Fragmentation

1. Take out the 10× Fragmentation Buffer, 5× Fragmentation Enzyme from KAPA HyperPlus kit stored at −20 °C, and thaw on ice.
2. Add 50 ng DNA in a final volume of 35 μL in low EDTA buffer to a 96-well plate placed in a plate chiller.
3. Set a thermal cycler on the following program and equilibrate for 5 min:

   37 °C 30 min

   4 °C HOLD

   Set heated lid to 47 °C.
4. Make the fragmentation mastermix as below allowing 10% extra if preparing for multiple samples, and mix well, spin down and place on ice.

Component	Volume (μL)
KAPA fragmentation buffer	5
KAPA fragmentation enzyme	10

5. Add 15 μL of Fragmentation mastermix to each sample while still on the plate chiller.
6. Seal the plate, invert to mix and centrifuge briefly.
7. Place the plate in the thermal cycler preset at 37 °C.
8. Fragment the DNA for 30 min to obtain fragments of 200–250 bp.
9. Replace the reagents at −20 °C.
10. When the incubation is complete centrifuge the plate briefly and transfer to a plate chiller.
11. *Optional: Remove 2 μL of each fragmented sample and run on the TapeStation with High Sensitivity reagents. Check that the mean peak size is 200–250 bp* (Fig. 1a). *Some optimization may be required depending on the DNA, thermal cycler and set-up conditions* (*see* **Note 4**).

3.3 End Repair and A-Tailing

1. Program a thermal cycler for the following conditions:

   65 °C 30 min

   4 °C HOLD

   Heated lid set to 75 °C

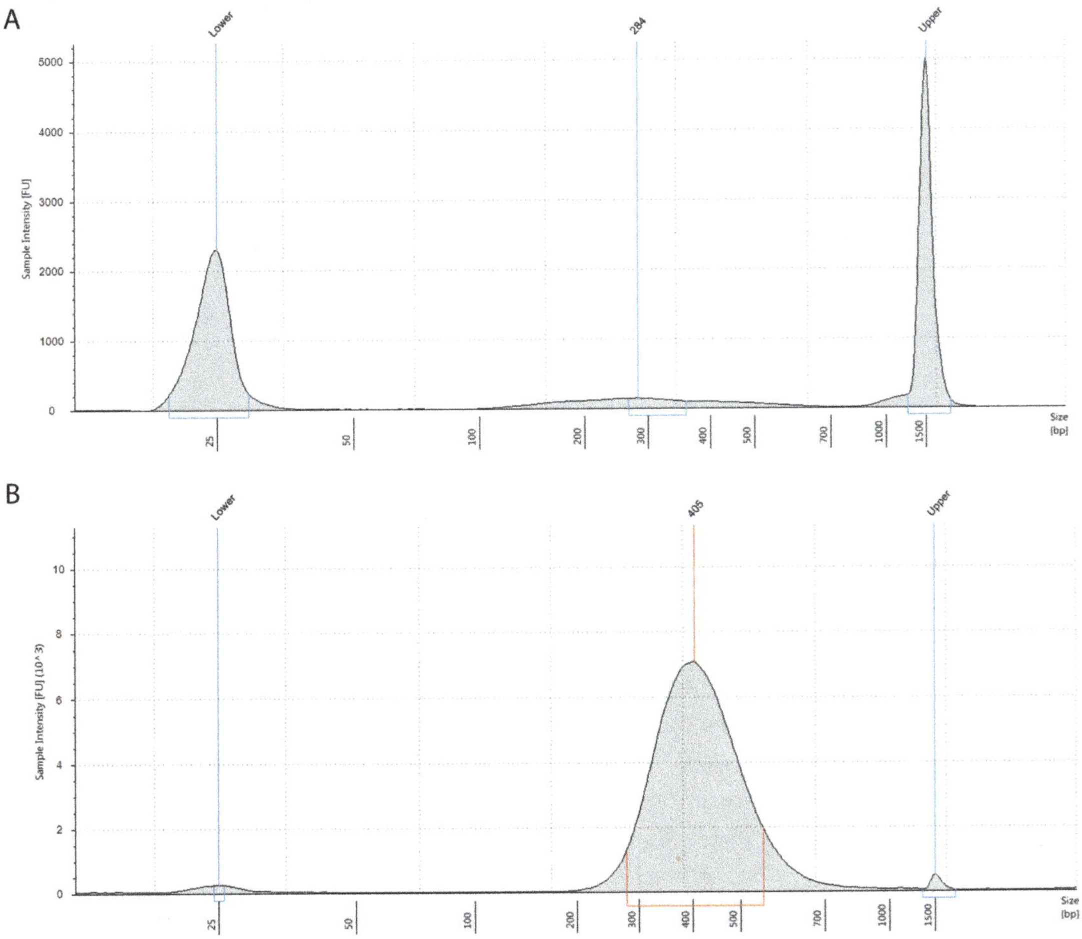

Fig. 1 (**a**) Fragmentation of genomic DNA should result in a peak around 200–250 bp (*see* Subheading 3.2, **step 11**). Visualized on the 2100 TapeStation (Agilent) High Sensitivity D100 ScreenTape). **(b)** Amplification of adapter ligated library should result in a peak ~400 bp (*see* Subheading 3.9, **step 2**). Visualized on the 2100 TapeStation (Agilent) High Sensitivity D100 ScreenTape

2. Thaw End Repair and A-tailing Buffer and enzyme mix and place on ice.
3. Vortex A-tailing buffer thoroughly to resuspend. Make sure all precipitates have disappeared.
4. Prepare a mastermix for the A-tailing reagents as follows, allowing 10% extra for pipetting error:

Component	Volume (μL)
End-repair and A-tailing buffer	7
End-repair and A-tailing enzyme	3

5. Vortex the mix, centrifuge briefly and add 10 μL of mastermix to each sample on the 96-well plate changing tips between each sample.
6. Seal the plate, invert several times to mix and centrifuge briefly.
7. Place the plate in the thermal cycler and incubate for 30 min at 65 °C.
8. When the program is completed, proceed immediately to the next step. Spin the plate briefly and place in a plate chiller.
9. Replace the reagents in −20 °C and proceed directly to adapter ligation (*see* **Note 5**).

3.4 Adapter Ligation

1. *For the first time use of the lyophilized SeqCap EZ Adapters, spin tubes and resuspend in 50 μL PCR-grade water. Mark with "R" as resuspended, vortex and spin down.*
2. Program a thermal cycler for the following conditions:

   20 °C 20 min

   4 °C HOLD

   Heated lid set to 37 °C
3. Take out Ligation Buffer and DNA Ligase and thaw on ice.
4. Vortex ligation buffer thoroughly to resuspended any precipitants.
5. Thaw SeqCap EZ Adapters used on ice. Each sample in the same pool must have different adapter. Use as many different adaptors as possible to allow for flexibility in multiplexing samples for sequencing. Note which sample receives which adapter.
6. Set up the Adapter Ligation mastermix as follows, allowing 10% extra for pipetting errors:

Component	Volume (μL)
PCR-grade water	2.5
Ligation buffer	30
DNA ligase	10

7. Vortex adapter ligation mastermix and centrifuge briefly.
8. Add 7.5 μL of resuspended SeqCap EZ adaptor to sample.
9. Add 42.5 μL of adapter ligation mastermix to each sample.
10. Seal the plate, invert several times to mix and centrifuge briefly.
11. Incubate the plate in the thermal cycler at 20 °C for 20 min.
12. Replace the buffer and enzyme mix in −20 °C.

3.5 Postligation Cleanup

1. Allow AMPure beads to warm to RT for 30 min. Vortex to resuspend fully.
2. Place the ligation plate in a plate adapter and remove the seal.
3. Add 88 μL of AMPure beads to each well.
4. Seal the plate securely and shake to mix the ligation reaction and the beads (*see* **Note 6**). Centrifuge the plate briefly. The beads should still be fully suspended after centrifugation.
5. Incubate samples at room temperature for 10 min.
6. Make fresh 80% EtOH by adding 40 mL 100% EtOH to 10 mL PCR-grade water. Empty the 80% EtOH into a disposable reservoir. Fresh 80% EtOH should always be used.
7. Place the plate on a magnetic stand. Allow 5 min for the beads to clear.
8. Using a multi-channel pipette remove as much as possible of the liquid without disturbing the beads (*see* **Note 7**).
9. Repeat the following steps THREE times using a multi-channel pipette (use fresh tips for each column of samples):
   (a) Add 200 μL fresh 80% EtOH to each well while on the magnet.
   (b) Remove the liquid without disturbing the beads and discard.
10. After THREE washes with 200 μL EtOH remove the remaining EtOH carefully with a 10 μL pipette tip.
11. Leave the plate open to dry at room temperature on the magnet for 10 min. Do not leave beads to dry for longer.
12. After 10 min remove the plate from the magnet and add 52 μL EB to the beads.
13. Seal the plate and mix to resuspend the beads. Spin briefly. Incubate for 2 min.
14. Place the plate on a magnetic stand for 5 min to allow the beads to clear.
15. Transfer 50 μL to a new labeled 96-well plate (*see* **Note 7**).

SAFE STOPPING POINT. Samples can be placed at 4 °C or at −20 °C for up to 72 h after elution.

3.6 Dual-SPRI Size Selection

1. Allow AMPure beads to warm to RT for 30 min. Vortex to resuspend fully.
2. Add 35 μL AMPure to each well containing sample.
3. Seal the plate, mix thoroughly by inverting and centrifuge briefly.
4. Incubate at RT for 15 min.

5. Place the plate on a magnetic stand for 2 min to allow the beads to clear.
6. Remove a total of 80 μL supernatant (*see* **Note 7**) to a new labeled plate without disturbing the beads. **Do not discard the supernatant.**
7. Add 10 μL AMPure to each well containing the 80 μL from the previous step.
8. Seal the plate, invert to mix, and centrifuge briefly.
9. Incubate at RT for 15 min.
10. Place the plate on a magnetic stand for 5 min to allow the beads to clear.
11. Remove the liquid without disturbing the beads (*see* **Note 7**) and discard.
12. Repeat the following steps THREE times using a multi-channel pipette (use fresh tips for each column of samples):
    (a) Add 200 μL fresh 80% EtOH to each tube while on the magnet.
    (b) Remove the liquid without disturbing the beads and discard.
13. After THREE washes with 200 μL EtOH remove remaining EtOH carefully with a 10 μL pipette tip.
14. Leave the plate open to dry at room temperature on the magnet for 10 min. Do not leave beads to dry for longer.
15. Remove the plate from the magnet and add 22 μL EB to the beads, seal the plate and invert few times to resuspend the beads.
16. Briefly centrifuge the plate and place it on a magnetic stand for 5 min to allow the beads to clear.
17. Transfer 20 μL of the samples to a new 96-well plate, using two transfers of 10 μL to avoid disturbing the beads.

SAFE STOPPING POINT. Samples can be placed at 4 °C or at −20 °C for up to 72 h after elution.

3.7 Library Amplification

1. For first time use, resuspend the SeqCap EZ "Pre-LM-PCR oligos 1 & 2" by spinning the tube and adding 550 μL PCR-grade water, vortex, spin down and place on ice. Mark the tube as resuspended "R".
2. Set up the Library Amplification mastermix as follows, allowing 10% extra for pipetting errors:

Component	Volume (μL)
HiFI HotStart ready mix	25
Library amplification primer mix	5

3. Vortex the mix and centrifuge briefly.
4. Add 30 μL of mastermix to each 20 μL sample.
5. Seal the 96-well plate, invert several times to mix and centrifuge briefly.
6. Place the 96-well plate in a thermal cycler and run the following program:

   Step 1: 98 °C 45 s

   Step 2: 98 °C 15 s

   Step 3: 60 °C 30 s

   Step 4: 72 °C 30 s

   Step 5: Repeat **steps 2–4** for a total of 6 cycles

   Step 6: 72 °C 1 min

   Step 7: 4 °C HOLD

   Heated lid set to 105 °C

SAFE STOPPING POINT. Samples can be placed at 4 °C or at -20 °C for up to 72 h after elution.

3.8 PCR Cleanup

1. Remove the Tapestation High Sensitivity reagents and Qubit standards from the fridge (if needed) and let them equilibrate to RT.
2. Allow the SeqCap EZ Purification beads to warm up to RT for 30 min. Vortex to resuspend fully.
3. Place the library amplification plate on a stand and add 50 μL DNA purification beads to the wells.
4. Seal the plate and invert to fully resuspend the beads.
5. Spin the plate briefly.
6. Incubate at RT for 15 min.
7. Make up fresh 80% EtOH by adding 40 mL EtOH to 10 mL PCR-grade water. Empty this into a disposable reservoir.
8. Place the plate on the magnetic stand. Allow 5 min to allow the beads to clear.
9. Remove the liquid without disturbing the beads using a multichannel pipette and two transfers of 90 μL and 10 μL (*see* **Note 7**).
10. Repeat the following steps THREE times using a multi-channel pipette (use fresh tips for each column of samples):
    (a) Add 200 μL fresh 80% EtOH to each tube while on the magnet.
    (b) Remove the liquid without disturbing the beads and discard.

11. After THREE washes with 200 μL EtOH remove remaining EtOH carefully with a 10 μL pipette tip.
12. Leave the plate open to dry at room temperature on the magnet for 10 min. Do not leave beads to dry for longer.
13. Remove the plate from the magnet and add 52 μL PCR-grade water to the beads.
14. Seal the plate, remove from the magnet, and mix to fully resuspend the beads.
15. Spin the plate briefly, and place back on the magnet.
16. Wait 5 min for the beads to clear.
17. Transfer 50 μL to a new plate using two transfers of 40 μL + 10μL to avoid disturbing the beads (*see* **Note** 7).
18. After removing sufficient volume for Tapestation and Qubit seal the plate.

3.9 Tapestation QC of Purified Amplified Library (Optional)

1. Remove 2 μL of each sample and run on the Tapestation High Sensitivity reagents.
2. Record the average fragment size between 50 and 900 bp which should be ~400 bp (Fig. 1b). No sharp peaks below 150 bp should be visible. Peaks <150 bp will most likely be adapter dimers resulting from inefficient washing of the PCR products. To remove adapter dimer peaks the number of ethanol washes in 3.8.10 may be increased to six.

3.10 Qubit of Purified Amplified Library

1. Quantify sample DNA concentrations using the HS Qubit reagents.
2. Record the values in ng/μL. Amplification with 6 cycles should yield >500 ng of library.

3.11 Preparation of Multiplex DNA Sample Pool

1. Before starting the process put heating block to 95 °C.
2. Start a thermal cycler set with a HOLD at 47 °C and the heated lid set to 57 °C.
3. For first time use, take out the SeqCap EZ HE-Oligos from SeqCap HE Oligo Kit A and B Kits and spin briefly:
   - Add 300 μL PCR-grade water to SeqCap EZ HE Universal Oligo Tube and vortex (400 μM).
   - Add 100 μL PCR-grade water to each SeqCap HE Index Oligo Tube and vortex (100 μM).
   - Mark the tubes as resuspended with a "R" on the tube.
4. Amplified indexed samples may be pooled prior to hybridization. Up to 10 samples have been reliably pooled. Each hybridization pool should contain a total of 1000 ng of DNA. This 1000 ng should be distributed equally between all samples

(i.e., if 10 samples use 100 ng of each) and each sample should have a different index adapter. Tumor and control samples from the same patient should be pooled together to minimize sequencing differences.

5. Remove required amount of DNA per sample for hybridization into a 1.5 mL tube, e.g., 100 ng if 10 samples are pooled. The total amount of DNA should be 1000 ng.
6. Seal the pre-hyb PCR plate with adhesive film. Freeze at −20 °C. These un-pooled libraries may be used for whole genome sequencing (WGS) by quantifying the library according to Subheading 3.16 and sequencing them directly on an Illumina sequencer. Depending on the depth of sequencing performed this can be useful for detection of non-coding variants (>40× sequencing depth) or for copy number analysis (0.1× sequencing depth, or ultra-low depth WGS).
7. To the tube with the pooled DNA add HE blocking oligos. For each 100 ng of DNA library used 1 μL of 100 μM Seqcap HE Index Oligo must be used. The blocking oligo number should match the ones used in the pool. For example, if four samples are pooled with indexes 2, 4, 6 and 8 the following amounts would be used:

Component	Amount of library used (total = 1000 ng)	Amount of HE Index Oligo (100 μM) required
SeqCap HE index 2 Oligo	250 ng	2.5 μL
SeqCap HE index 4 Oligo	250 ng	2.5 μL
SeqCap HE index 6 Oligo	250 ng	2.5 μL
SeqCap HE index 8 Oligo	250 ng	2.5 μL

8. To the pooled DNA and HE-oligo mix add:

   2.5 μL of Universal HE oligo.

   5 μL of COT Human DNA.
9. Vortex and spin the tube(s) now containing the multiplex DNA sample libraries, COT DNA and the HE oligos.
10. Cover the open 1.5 mL tube with a piece of parafilm and pierce 4 small holes in the top with a pipette tip.
11. Place the tube in a SpeedVac on high heat (60 °C) until the tube is completely dry. Depending on the volume this takes 40–70 min.

3.12 Hybridization

1. Reagents are in SeqCap EZ Hybridization and Wash Kit.
2. Equilibrate a thermocycler to 47 °C with the heated lid set to 57 °C.
3. Remove the parafilm from the DNA pool tube. Add to the tube:

Component	Volume (μL)
2× hybridization buffer (vial 5)	7.5
Hybridization component A (vial 6)	3.0

4. Close the tube and vortex for 10 s.
5. Centrifuge at maximum speed for 10 s.
6. Place the hybridization mix in a hot block at 95 °C for 10 min to denature the DNA. Place a weight on top of the tube to prevent it popping open.
7. To a 0.2 mL strip tube for hybridization add (prepare a separate 0.2 mL tube for each pool) 4.5 μL EZ Library for each pool (*see* **Note 8**).
8. Place 2 strips of empty tubes down the sides of the thermocycler to prevent crushing of the sample tubes.
9. When the hybridization mix has completed the 10 min denaturation, quickly spin the 1.5 mL tube and transfer all the volume to the prepared 0.2 mL tube with EZ library and water.
10. Close the 0.2 mL tube and incubate in the preset thermocycler at 47 °C for *at least* 16 h.

3.13 Hybridization Cleanup

1. Take out the Post-LM-PCR oligos 1 & 2 and KAPA HiFi Hotstart ready mix and place them on ice. (Reagents in SeqCap EZ Accessory Kit v.2).
2. Thaw hybridization wash buffers at RT for 5–10 min.
3. Add PCR-grade water to the buffers:

   (a) To 40 μL of 10× Stringent Wash Buffer add 360 μL of PCR-grade water.

   Aliquot 1× Stringent Wash Buffer into 2 × 200 μL in 0.2 mL strip tubes.

   Place in thermal cycler for 2 h with temperature set at 47 °C and heated.

   Lid at 57 °C.

   (b) To 30 μL 10× Wash Buffer I add 270 μL of PCR-grade water.

Aliquot 1× Wash Buffer I 1 × 100 μL in 0.2 mL strip tubes.

Place in thermal cycler 2 h with temperature set at 47 °C and heated.

Lid at 57 °C and set volume to 200 μL.

Leave remaining 200 μL in the 1.5 mL tube at RT.

(c) To 20 μL 10× Wash Buffer II add 180 μL of PCR-grade water.

Leave the tube at RT.

(d) To 20 μL 10× Wash Buffer III add 180 μL of PCR-grade water.

Leave the tube at RT.

(e) To 200 μL 2.5× Bead Wash Buffer add 300 μL of PCR-grade water.

Leave the tube at RT.

4. Take out the Capture Beads from the Pure Capture Bead Kit allow them to equilibrate to RT for 30 min.
5. One hour after placing 1× Stringent Wash Buffers and 1× Wash Buffer I to 47 °C proceed to washing the Capture Beads.
6. Vortex the beads to resuspend.
7. Aliquot 100 μL of beads per capture pool into a 0.2 mL tube.
8. Place the tube in a magnetic stand and allow the liquid to clear, approximately for 1 min.
9. Remove and discard the liquid.
10. Remove the tube from the magnet.
11. Repeat **steps a-e** twice:
    (a) Add 200 μL of 1× Bead Wash Buffer, close the tube.
    (b) Vortex and spin down briefly.
    (c) Place the tube in a magnet stand and allow the liquid to clear.
    (d) Remove and discard the liquid.
    (e) Remove the tube from the magnet
12. Add 100 μL of 1× Bead Wash Buffer, close the tube.
13. Vortex and spin down briefly.
14. Place the tube on the magnet.
15. Remove and discard the liquid and ***immediately proceed*** to adding the pool. ***Do not let the beads dry!***

16. Remove the hybridized pool samples from the thermocycler and spin briefly.
17. Transfer the entire pool, 15 μL, to the prepared beads. Mix by pipetting.
18. Close the tube and place in a thermocycler at 47 °C for 15 min.
19. Remove the tube, vortex, spin briefly and place back in the thermocycler for 15 min.
20. Remove the tube, vortex, spin briefly and place back in the thermocycler for 15 min.
21. Remove the tube, add 100 μL preheated 1× Wash Buffer I to the beads.
22. Mix by pipetting ten times.
23. Place the tube in a magnet stand and allow the liquid to clear.
24. Remove and discard the liquid.
25. Repeat **steps 1–6** twice:
    (a) Remove the tube from the magnet.
    (b) Add 200 μL of preheated 1× Stringent Wash Buffer, close the tube.
    (c) Vortex and spin down briefly.
    (d) Place the tube in the thermocycler at 47°C for 5 min.
    (e) Place the tube in a magnet stand and allow the liquid to clear.
    (f) Remove and discard the liquid.
26. Remove the tube from the magnet.
27. Add 200 μL of RT 1× Wash Buffer I, close the tube.
28. Vortex for 2 min and spin down briefly.
29. Place the tube in a magnet stand for 3 min or until liquid is clear.
30. Remove and discard the liquid.
31. Remove the tube from the magnet.
32. Add 200 μL of RT 1× Wash Buffer II, close the tube.
33. Vortex for 1 min and spin down briefly.
34. Place the tube in a magnet stand for 5 min or until liquid is clear.
35. Remove and discard the liquid.
36. Remove the tube from the magnet.
37. Add 200 μL of RT 1× Wash Buffer III, close the tube.
38. Vortex for 30 s and spin down briefly.

39. Place the tube in a magnet stand for 5 min or until liquid is clear.
40. Remove all liquid in two steps by first removing 180 μL and subsequently 20 μL with a small pipette tip.
41. Remove the tube from the magnet.
42. Add 40 μL of PCR-grade water to the beads.
43. Vortex and spin down briefly.
44. Store on ice until used.

3.14 Amplify the Captured Multiplex Pool

1. Place a 96- well optical plate on a chiller.
2. Set up the Post-capture Pool Amplification mastermix as below. Two reactions are needed per hybridized pool.

Component	Volume (μL)
KAPA HiFi HotStart ReadyMix (2×)	25
Post-LM-PCR Oligos 1 & 2 (5 μM)	5

3. Vortex the mix, and spin briefly.
4. Set up 2 reactions per pool in a 96-well plate:
   (a) Pipette 30 μL of mastermix into two wells per pool.
   (b) Pipette 20 μL of pool/bead slurry into two wells per pool.
5. Seal the plate, mix by inverting and centrifuge briefly.
6. Place in a thermocycler using the following program:

   Step 1: 45 s 98 °C

   Step 2: 15 s 98 °C

   Step 3: 30 s 60 °C

   Step 4: 30 s 72 °C

   Step 5: Go to **step 2**, repeat ten times

   Step 6: 1 min 72 °C

   Step 7: HOLD 4 °C

SAFE STOPPING POINT. After the PCR the plate can be left on the cycler at 4 °C or at −20 °C.

3.15 Post-PCR Cleanup of Amplified Capture Pool

1. In Pre-PCR allow the SeqCap EZ Purification beads from the Nimblegen kit to warm to RT for 30 min.
2. Vortex to resuspend fully.
3. Aliquot 180 μL DNA purification beads per pool into 1.5 mL tubes and take to Post-PCR room.
4. Open the plate containing the amplified library and pipette 90 μL of SeqCap EZ Purification beads into each well.
5. Seal the plate and mix. Spin briefly.
6. Incubate at RT for 15 min.
7. Make up fresh 80% EtOH by adding 40 mL 100% EtOH to 10 mL PCR-grade water and empty into a disposable reservoir.
8. After 15 min incubation place the plate on a magnetic stand for 5 min to allow the beads to clear.
9. Remove the liquid without disturbing the beads.
10. Repeat **steps 1–3** twice:
    (a) Add 200 μL fresh 80% EtOH to each well while on the magnet.
    (b) Leave for 30 s.
    (c) Remove the liquid without disturbing the beads.
11. Remove remaining EtOH with 10 μL pipette.
12. Leave the samples to dry on the magnet for 15 min.
13. Remove the plate from the magnet and add 26 μL PCR-grade water to the beads.
14. Seal the plate and resuspend by mixing and spin briefly.
15. Incubate at RT for 2 min.
16. Place the plate on a magnetic stand for 5 min to allow the beads to clear.
17. Transfer 25 μL of the cleaned up reaction into the labeled 1.5 mL lo-bind tube, combining the two PCR reactions from the same Pool in one tube.
18. Remove 2 μL of each pool and run on the TapeStation High Sensitivity reagents.
19. Record the average fragment size between 50 and 900 bp.

SAFE STOPPING POINT. Store the pool at –20° C.

3.16 qPCR of Amplified Pool Prep

1. For first time use of KAPA Library Quantification Kit add 1 mL Illumina Primer premix to the 5 mL bottle of KAPA SYBR FAST qPCR mix and vortex. Mark the bottle to indicate primers have been added.
2. Remove the KAPA Library Quantification kit from the freezer and allow defrosting.

3. Prepare the following dilutions of the libraries **in Post-PCR** into 1.5 mL lo-bind tubes for each pool:
   (a) Add 999 μL of PCR-grade water into a tube labeled with 1/1000 diln (1) and the unique pool number.
   (b) Add 90 μL of PCR-grade water into a tube labeled with 1/10000 diln (2) and the unique pool number.
   (c) Add 50 μL of PCR-grade water into a tube labeled with 1/20000 diln (3) and the unique pool number.
   (d) To the tube containing 999 μL of water add 1 μL of purified pool. Close and vortex.
   (e) To the tube containing 90 μL of water add 10 μL of the first dilution (1). Close and vortex.
   (f) To the tube containing 50 μL of water add 50 μL of the second dilution (2). Close and vortex.
   (g) Discard the 1/1000 dilution as this will not be used.
4. **In Pre-PCR** prepare the KAPA post-hyb qPCR mastermix in a 1.5 mL lo-bind tube. Enough mix is needed for six standards, pool dilutions 2 and 3, and NTC in duplicate.

Component	Volume (μL)
KAPA SYBR FAST qPCR mix	12
ROX low[a]	0.4
Water	3.6

[a]ROX Low or ROX High can be used depending on the qPCR machine. Check the compatibility for specific qPCR machines

5. Set up a Fast Optical 96-well plate with standards, NTC and pool dilutions in duplicate.
6. Add 16 μL of mastermix to each well.
7. Add 4 μL of each KAPA standard to the plate.
8. Add 4 μL of pool dilutions 2 and 3 to the plate.
9. Add 4 μL of PCR-grade water to the NTC wells.
10. Seal the plate with an optical film and invert the plate to mix and spin down.
11. Place the plate into the 7500 Fast real-time machine, or equivalent, and run in fast mode for SYBR green.
12. When the run has completed select any empty wells on the plate, right click and select "Omit." Press "Analyze" to reanalyze the data.
13. Check the standard curve has an R squared >0.9 by clicking on Standard Curve and highlighting all wells.

14. Determine the average concentration for each pool by comparing values against the standard curve. Multiply by the dilution factor and adjust for the average size of the amplified library (from Subheading 3.15) against the size of the products in the standard curve (452 bp) to determine the molarity of the library.
15. The library is ready for sequencing on any Illumina-based sequencer. Depending on the purpose, somewhere between 100 and 250× coverage is recommended. Paired-end reads should also be performed to enable detection of translocations.

4 Notes

1. To remove EDTA in DNA solutions either a column-based reextraction of DNA or ethanol precipitation can be performed. For column reextraction (e.g., DNA Clean & Concentrator-5) use 2 volumes of DNA binding buffer per volume of genomic DNA. After washing elute the DNA in low EDTA buffer such as EB. For ethanol precipitation of DNA add 0.1 volumes of 3 M NaAc and 2.5 volumes of cold 100% ethanol to genomic DNA. Mix well, spin briefly and place on ice for 30 min. Centrifuge at maximum speed (>13,000 × *g*) in a benchtop centrifuge for 15 min. Immediately remove from centrifuge and aspirate supernatant, being careful not to remove the DNA pellet. Add 200 μL 70% ethanol, centrifuge for 5 min and aspirate supernatant. Leave to dry. Resuspend DNA in appropriate volume of low EDTA buffer.
2. To concentrate DNA take the sample tube and cover the top with parafilm. Pierce four holes in the parafilm using a 10 μL pipette tip. Place the tube in the concentrator (with a balance) and set the temperature to (off). Start the concentrator and check periodically until the volume has reduced sufficiently to adjust the concentration to >4 ng/μL. If the volume is reduced too much resuspend the DNA in the original elution solution. Once concentrated remove the tube from the concentrator, remove the parafilm and close the tube. Vortex the tube well to resuspend any DNA which may have pelleted, and spin the tube. Requantify the DNA using the Qubit as before
3. If the DNA concentration is >50 ng/μL the DNA should be diluted for use. Remove enough DNA from the stock tube for the purpose, plus a little extra to allow for requantification. Dilute the DNA in low EDTA buffer such as EB. Once diluted, requantify the DNA using HS Qubit and use this value to calculate the volume of DNA required for the assay.

4. If DNA fragments are outside of the recommended range after fragmentation the incubation time can be modified. If smaller fragments are required increase the incubation time, and if larger fragments are required the incubation time can be shortened. The most likely cause of inconsistent fragment sizes is EDTA in the DNA elution buffer. EDTA interferes with the fragmentation enzyme. This can be overcome either by repurifying the DNA or using the conditioning buffer in the HyperPlus kit, which chelates the EDTA. Optimization for DNA eluted in different buffers will be required.
5. It is important to proceed directly to adapter ligation once A-tailing has completed in order to maximize ligation efficiency. If samples are left overnight or stored at −20 °C the A-tails may fall off resulting in failure to ligate the adapters, decreased library complexity and an increase in duplicate reads.
6. The adapter Ligation reaction is very viscose and it is important to mix the solution thoroughly to ensure the beads are homogenous and bind the DNA efficiently.
7. Bead cleanup. During bead cleanup it is important to ensure that beads are not transferred with the removal of buffer. To prevent carryover it is easier to remove the supernatant using two transfers where the last volume is 10 μL. For example, when removing the ligation mix from the beads transfer 190 μL followed by removal of the final 10 μL using a small tip.
8. The Seqcap EZ probe library should be aliquoted before use to prevent degradation due to freeze–thaw cycles. Thaw the probe library on ice, vortex and spin briefly. Aliquot the probe library into 4.5 μL single use aliquots in 0.2 mL tubes and store at −20 °C until needed.

References

1. Morgan GJ, Walker BA, Davies FE (2012) The genetic architecture of multiple myeloma. Nat Rev Cancer 12(5):335–348. https://doi.org/10.1038/nrc3257
2. Boyd KD, Ross FM, Chiecchio L, Dagrada G, Konn ZJ, Tapper WJ, Walker BA, Wardell CP, Gregory WM, Szubert AJ, Bell SE, Child JA, Jackson GH, Davies FE, Morgan GJ (2012) A novel prognostic model in myeloma based on co-segregating adverse FISH lesions and the ISS: analysis of 1180 patients treated in the MRC myeloma IX trial. Leukemia 26(2):349–355
3. Shaughnessy J, Hanamura I, Burington B, Sawyer J, Crowley J, Barlogie B (2005) Interphase FISH-defined amplification of chromosome 1q21 (AMP1q21) identify high-risk subsets among patients with multiple myeloma (MM) lacking metaphase cytogenetic abnormalities (CA). Blood 106(11):185a
4. Chiecchio L, Dagrada GP, Protheroe RK, Stockley DM, Smith AG, Orchard KH, Cross NC, Harrison CJ, Ross FM (2009) Loss of 1p and rearrangement of MYC are associated with progression of smouldering myeloma to myeloma: sequential analysis of a single case. Haematologica 94(7):1024–1028. https://doi.org/10.3324/haematol.2008.004440
5. Chiecchio L, Protheroe RK, Ibrahim AH, Cheung KL, Rudduck C, Dagrada GP, Cabanas ED, Parker T, Nightingale M, Wechalekar A, Orchard KH, Harrison CJ, Cross NC, Morgan GJ, Ross FM (2006) Deletion of chromosome

13 detected by conventional cytogenetics is a critical prognostic factor in myeloma. Leukemia 20:1610–1617

6. Ross FM, Avet-Loiseau H, Ameye G, Gutierrez NC, Liebisch P, O'Connor S, Dalva K, Fabris S, Testi AM, Jarosova M, Hodkinson C, Collin A, Kerndrup G, Kuglik P, Ladon D, Bernasconi P, Maes B, Zemanova Z, Michalova K, Michau L, Neben K, Hermansen NE, Rack K, Rocci A, Protheroe R, Chiecchio L, Poirel HA, Sonneveld P, Nyegaard M, Johnsen HE, European Myeloma N (2012) Report from the European myeloma network on interphase FISH in multiple myeloma and related disorders. Haematologica 97(8):1272–1277. https://doi.org/10.3324/haematol.2011.056176
7. Walker BA, Boyle EM, Wardell CP, Murison A, Begum DB, Dahir NM, Proszek PZ, Johnson DC, Kaiser MF, Melchor L, Aronson LI, Scales M, Pawlyn C, Mirabella F, Jones JR, Brioli A, Mikulasova A, Cairns DA, Gregory WM, Quartilho A, Drayson MT, Russell N, Cook G, Jackson GH, Leleu X, Davies FE, Morgan GJ (2015) Mutational spectrum, copy number changes, and outcome: results of a sequencing study of patients with newly diagnosed myeloma. J Clin Oncol 33(33):3911–3920. https://doi.org/10.1200/JCO.2014.59.1503
8. Walker BA, Leone PE, Chiecchio L, Dickens NJ, Jenner MW, Boyd KD, Johnson DC, Gonzalez D, Dagrada GP, Protheroe RK, Konn ZJ, Stockley DM, Gregory WM, Davies FE, Ross FM, Morgan GJ (2010) A compendium of myeloma-associated chromosomal copy number abnormalities and their prognostic value. Blood 116(15):e56–e65. https://doi.org/10.1182/blood-2010-04-279596
9. Chapman MA, Lawrence MS, Keats JJ, Cibulskis K, Sougnez C, Schinzel AC, Harview CL, Brunet JP, Ahmann GJ, Adli M, Anderson KC, Ardlie KG, Auclair D, Baker A, Bergsagel PL, Bernstein BE, Drier Y, Fonseca R, Gabriel SB, Hofmeister CC, Jagannath S, Jakubowiak AJ, Krishnan A, Levy J, Liefeld T, Lonial S, Mahan S, Mfuko B, Monti S, Perkins LM, Onofrio R, Pugh TJ, Rajkumar SV, Ramos AH, Siegel DS, Sivachenko A, Stewart AK, Trudel S, Vij R, Voet D, Winckler W, Zimmerman T, Carpten J, Trent J, Hahn WC, Garraway LA, Meyerson M, Lander ES, Getz G, Golub TR (2011) Initial genome sequencing and analysis of multiple myeloma. Nature 471(7339):467–472. https://doi.org/10.1038/nature09837
10. Walker BA, Wardell CP, Melchor L, Hulkki S, Potter NE, Johnson DC, Fenwick K, Kozarewa I, Gonzalez D, Lord CJ, Ashworth A, Davies FE, Morgan GJ (2012) Intraclonal heterogeneity and distinct molecular mechanisms characterize the development of t(4;14) and t(11;14) myeloma. Blood 120(5):1077–1086. https://doi.org/10.1182/blood-2012-03-412981
11. Lohr JG, Stojanov P, Carter SL, Cruz-Gordillo P, Lawrence MS, Auclair D, Sougnez C, Knoechel B, Gould J, Saksena G, Cibulskis K, McKenna A, Chapman MA, Straussman R, Levy J, Perkins LM, Keats JJ, Schumacher SE, Rosenberg M, Multiple Myeloma Research C, Getz G, Golub TR (2014) Widespread genetic heterogeneity in multiple myeloma: implications for targeted therapy. Cancer Cell 25(1):91–101. https://doi.org/10.1016/j.ccr.2013.12.015
12. Bolli N, Avet-Loiseau H, Wedge DC, Van Loo P, Alexandrov LB, Martincorena I, Dawson KJ, Iorio F, Nik-Zainal S, Bignell GR, Hinton JW, Li Y, Tubio JM, McLaren S, OM S, Butler AP, Teague JW, Mudie L, Anderson E, Rashid N, Tai YT, Shammas MA, Sperling AS, Fulciniti M, Richardson PG, Parmigiani G, Magrangeas F, Minvielle S, Moreau P, Attal M, Facon T, Futreal PA, Anderson KC, Campbell PJ, Munshi NC (2014) Heterogeneity of genomic evolution and mutational profiles in multiple myeloma. Nat Commun 5:2997. https://doi.org/10.1038/ncomms3997
13. Melchor L, Brioli A, Wardell CP, Murison A, Potter NE, Kaiser MF, Fryer RA, Johnson DC, Begum DB, Hulkki Wilson S, Vijayaraghavan G, Titley I, Cavo M, Davies FE, Walker BA, Morgan GJ (2014) Single-cell genetic analysis reveals the composition of initiating clones and phylogenetic patterns of branching and parallel evolution in myeloma. Leukemia 28(8):1705–1715. https://doi.org/10.1038/leu.2014.13
14. Walker BA, Wardell CP, Murison A, Boyle EM, Begum DB, Dahir NM, Proszek PZ, Melchor L, Pawlyn C, Kaiser MF, Johnson DC, Qiang YW, Jones JR, Cairns DA, Gregory WM, Owen RG, Cook G, Drayson MT, Jackson GH, Davies FE, Morgan GJ (2015) APOBEC family mutational signatures are associated with poor prognosis translocations in multiple myeloma. Nat Commun 6:6997. https://doi.org/10.1038/ncomms7997
15. Weinhold N, Ashby C, Rasche L, Chavan SS, Stein C, Stephens OW, Tytarenko R, Bauer MA, Meissner T, Deshpande S, Patel PH, Buzder T, Molnar G, Peterson EA, van Rhee F, Zangari M, Thanendrarajan S, Schinke C, Tian E, Epstein J, Barlogie B, Davies FE, Heuck CJ, Walker BA, Morgan GJ (2016) Clonal selection and double hit events involving tumor suppressor genes underlie relapse from chemotherapy: myeloma as a model. Blood

128(13):1735–1744. https://doi.org/10.1182/blood-2016-06-723007

16. Walker BA, Leone PE, Jenner MW, Li C, Gonzalez D, Johnson DC, Ross FM, Davies FE, Morgan GJ (2006) Integration of global SNP-based mapping and expression arrays reveals key regions, mechanisms and genes important in the pathogenesis of multiple myeloma. Blood 108(5):1733–1743
17. Walker BA, Morgan GJ (2006) Use of single nucleotide polymorphism-based mapping arrays to detect copy number changes and loss of heterozygosity in multiple myeloma. Clin Lymphoma Myeloma 7(3):186–191
18. Chesi M, Bergsagel PL, Brents LA, Smith CM, Gerhard DS, Kuehl WM (1996) Dysregulation of cyclin D1 by translocation into an IgH gamma switch region in two multiple myeloma cell lines. Blood 88(2):674–681
19. Chesi M, Nardini E, Brents LA, Schrock E, Ried T, Kuehl WM, Bergsagel PL (1997) Frequent translocation t(4;14)(p16.3;q32.3) in multiple myeloma is associated with increased expression and activating mutations of fibroblast growth factor receptor 3. Nat Genet 16(3):260–264
20. Nishida K, Tamura A, Nakazawa N, Ueda Y, Abe T, Matsuda F, Kashima K, Taniwaki M (1997) The Ig heavy chain gene is frequently involved in chromosomal translocations in multiple myeloma and plasma cell leukemia as detected by in situ hybridization. Blood 90(2):526–534
21. Lieber MR (2016) Mechanisms of human lymphoid chromosomal translocations. Nat Rev Cancer 16(6):387–398. https://doi.org/10.1038/nrc.2016.40
22. Walker BA, Wardell CP, Johnson DC, Kaiser MF, Begum DB, Dahir NB, Ross FM, Davies FE, Gonzalez D, Morgan GJ (2013) Characterization of IGH locus breakpoints in multiple myeloma indicates a subset of translocations appear to occur in pregerminal center B cells. Blood 121(17):3413–3419. https://doi.org/10.1182/blood-2012-12-471888
23. Walker BA, Wardell CP, Brioli A, Boyle E, Kaiser MF, Begum DB, Dahir NB, Johnson DC, Ross FM, Davies FE, Morgan GJ (2014) Translocations at 8q24 juxtapose MYC with genes that harbor superenhancers resulting in overexpression and poor prognosis in myeloma patients. Blood Cancer J 4:e191. https://doi.org/10.1038/bcj.2014.13
24. Affer M, Chesi M, Chen WD, Keats JJ, Demchenko YN, Tamizhmani K, Garbitt VM, Riggs DL, Brents LA, Roschke AV, Van Wier S, Fonseca R, Bergsagel PL, Kuehl WM (2014) Promiscuous MYC locus rearrangements hijack enhancers but mostly super-enhancers to dysregulate MYC expression in multiple myeloma. Leukemia 28(8):1725–1735. https://doi.org/10.1038/leu.2014.70

Chapter 7

RNA-Sequencing from Low-Input Material in Multiple Myeloma for Application in Clinical Routine

Anja Seckinger, Tomi Bähr-Ivacevic, Vladimir Benes, and Dirk Hose

Abstract

RNA sequencing is a recently developed approach for transcriptome profiling with several advantages over gene expression profiling using DNA microarrays. Here we describe a RNA-sequencing protocol optimized for low-input analysis of total RNA from CD138+ purified plasma cells from myeloma patients which is applicable in clinical routine.

Key words Multiple myeloma, RNA-sequencing, Low input, Clinical application

1 Introduction

Malignant plasma cells from patients with multiple myeloma harbor a high median number of chromosomal aberrations and multiple changes in gene expression compared to normal bone marrow plasma cells [1–8].

During the last 15 years, the gene expression profile of CD138+ purified myeloma cells was assessed most often by using Affymetrix U133 2.0 microarrays. It can be performed and reported in clinical routine within 4–6 weeks using our (free) open-source software-framework GEP-R including our HM-metascore [9] in >80% of patients as we have shown for our GMMG-MM5 phase III clinical trial. Gene expression analysis allows (i) simultaneously assessing the expression of (almost) all genes, without the need of a preselection of interesting genes or regions, (ii) risk stratification [10–12], (iii) performing a molecular classification grouping multiple myeloma into different subentities [13, 14], (iv) assessing surrogates of biological variables, which in turn might also have prognostic relevance, such as proliferation [4], and (v) assessing expression of potential therapeutic targets (e.g., Aurora kinase A or B-cell maturation antigen [5, 15]).

Christoph Heuck and Niels Weinhold (eds.), *Multiple Myeloma: Methods and Protocols*, Methods in Molecular Biology, vol. 1792, https://doi.org/10.1007/978-1-4939-7865-6_7, © Springer Science+Business Media, LLC, part of Springer Nature 2018

RNA-sequencing (RNA-seq) is a recently developed approach for transcriptome profiling and has five main advantages over gene expression profiling using microarrays: (i) It provides quantification of levels of transcripts without significant saturation effects. (ii) It does not prerequisite a priori definition of sequences to be analyzed (as are for example Affymetrix "probesets") and thus allows for detection of mutated transcripts (e.g., BRAF-mutations [16]). Likewise, transcripts, for which initially incorrect sequences were assumed, and thus corresponding probesets do not interrogate the transcript of interest, can be analyzed. (iii) RNA-sequencing can routinely be performed successfully from as low input as 10 pg of total RNA (compared to about 100 ng for microarrays and a double amplification protocol). The latter is especially important for myeloma research, as in about 20% of patients the amount of material does not permit an analysis. (iv) RNA-sequencing enables the analysis of splice variants and (v) the investigation of other RNA types, e.g., miRNAs [17] (the latter needs specific protocols not included in this chapter).

Here we describe a RNA-sequencing protocol optimized for low-input analysis of purified malignant plasma cells applicable in clinical routine diagnostics.

2 Materials

The protocol for cDNA synthesis is theoretically applicable for starting from 10 pg of total RNA. However, we recommend to start with 1–5 ng of total RNA. Purified total RNA should be in nuclease-free water. We recommend evaluating total RNA-quantity, for example using a Qubit Fluorometer (Thermo Fisher Scientific), as well as RNA-quality, for example using an Agilent 2100 BioAnalyzer, before sequencing. The following kits have been optimized for this particular protocol. Their substitution or modifications of the protocol may lead to unexpected results. Thoroughly follow all waste disposal regulations when disposing waste materials.

1. SMARTer® Ultra Low RNA Kit for Illumina® Sequencing (Clontech Laboratories).
2. Agilent High Sensitivity DNA Kit (Agilent Technologies).
3. Qubit™ dsDNA HS Assay Kit (Thermo Fisher Scientific).
4. NEBNext® ChIP-Seq Library Prep Master Mix Set for Illumina® Sequencing (New England BioLabs).
5. SPRI AMPure XP Beads (Beckman Coulter).

3 Methods

3.1 First-Strand cDNA Synthesis

1. Using the SMARTer® Ultra Low RNA Kit for Illumina® Sequencing, prepare a stock solution of Reaction Buffer by mixing 19 μL of Dilution Buffer with 1 μL of RNase Inhibitor (*see* **Note 1**). Scale-up if needed.
2. Set up positive and negative controls (usually done if a new kit is used) as well as test samples (*see* Table 1). Transfer each whole volume of 3.5 μL to individual 0.2 mL RNase-free PCR tubes in an 8-well strip. Starting amount is commonly 5 ng of total RNA.
3. Place samples from **step 2** on a −20 °C prechilled PCR rack, add 1 μL of 3′ SMART CDS Primer II A (12 μM); total volume: 4.5 μL. Mix the contents gently and spin the tubes briefly in the microcentrifuge.
4. Incubate the tubes at 72 °C in a hot-lid thermal cycler for 3 min. Afterwards, put the samples on ice (*see* **Note 2**).
5. In the meantime, prepare a Master Mix for all reactions (plus an additional one as surplus) by combining the following reagents in the order shown, at room temperature to a total volume of 5.5 μL: 2 μL of 5× First-strand buffer, 0.25 μL of DTT (100 mM), 1 μL of dNTP Mix (10 mM), 1 μL of SMARTer IIA oligonucleotide (12 μM), 0.25 μL RNase inhibitor, and 1 μL of SMARTScribe reverse transcriptase (100 U). Gently vortex to mix and spin briefly in the microcentrifuge. Note: The reverse transcriptase should be added just prior to use.
6. Add 5.5 μL of the Master Mix to each reaction tube from **step 4**. Mix the contents of the tubes by gently pipetting, and spin the tubes briefly to collect the liquid at the bottom.

Table 1
Preparation of controls and test samples for cDNA synthesis

Components	Negative control (μL)	Positive control (μL)	Test sample (μL)
Reaction buffer	2.5	2.5	2.5
Nuclease-free water	1	–	–
Diluted control RNA[a]	–	1	–
Sample	–	–	1
Total volume	**3.5**	**3.5**	**3.5**

[a]Control RNA is supplied at a concentration of 1 μg/μL and should be diluted in nuclease-free water to match the concentration of the test sample

7. Incubate the tubes at 42 °C for 90 min.
8. Terminate the reaction by heating the tubes at 70 °C for 10 min.

3.2 Purification of First-Strand cDNA Using SPRI Ampure Beads

1. Bring beads to room temperature before use and mix to disperse completely.
2. Add 25 μL of SPRI Ampure XP beads to each sample. Mix thoroughly by pipetting the entire volume up and down (10×). As beads are viscous, suck up the entire volume and push it out slowly. To allow DNA binding to the beads, incubate at room temperature for 8 min.
3. Spin sample tubes briefly to collect the liquid at the bottom. Place the sample tubes on a magnetic separation device until the solution is completely clear (approx. 5 min).
4. While samples are still on the magnetic separation device, pipet out the solution and discard. Briefly spin the tubes to collect the liquid at the bottom.
5. Place the tubes back in a magnetic separation device to let beads separate from the liquid completely (approx. 2 min or longer). Pipet out the residual liquid from the beads using a 10 μL pipetman and discard. Make sure that there is no supernatant remaining in the tube. Note: Be careful not to take out any beads with the supernatant.

3.3 ds cDNA Amplification by Long-Distance PCR

1. Prepare a PCR Master Mix for all reactions (plus an additional one as surplus) by combining the following reagents in the order shown (total volume: 50 μL): 5 μL of 10× Advantage 2 PCR buffer, 2 μL of dNTP Mix (10 mM), 2 μL of IS PCR primer (12 μM), 2 μL of 50× Advantage 2 polymerase mix, 39 μL of nuclease-free water. Mix well by vortexing and spin the tube briefly in the microcentrifuge.
2. Add 50 μL of PCR Master Mix from **step 1** to each tube containing DNA bound to the beads from Subheading 3.2, **step 5**. Mix well and briefly spin down.
3. Place the tube in a preheated thermal cycler with a heated lid. Start thermal cycling using the following program:

   95 °C 1 min

   12 cycles*:

   - 95 °C 15 s
   - 65 °C 30 s
   - 68 °C 6 min

   72 °C 10 min

   10 °C ∞

*Note: The optimal number of cycles has to be determined; see the User Manual for details.

3.4 Purification of ds cDNA Using SPRI Ampure Beads

1. Cover all the wells of a 96-well V-bottom plate with a clean adhesive seal. Uncover only the wells that you want to use. Vortex SPRI beads until homogenously dispersed and add 90 μL of SPRI Ampure XP Beads to the uncovered 96-wells.
2. Transfer the entire PCR product including the SPRI beads from Subheading 3.3, **step 3** to the wells of the plate containing the SPRI beads from **step 1** above. Mix thoroughly by pipetting the entire volume up and down (10×). As beads are viscous, suck up the entire volume and push it out slowly. To allow DNA binding to the beads, incubate at room temperature for 8 min.
3. Place the 96-well plate on a magnetic stand until the liquid is completely clear and there are no beads left in the supernatant (approx. 5 min).
4. Pipet out the supernatant, while the plate is still sitting on the magnetic stand.
5. While the plate is on the magnetic stand, to wash away contaminants add 200 μL of freshly made 80% ethanol to each sample without disturbing the beads. Wait for 30 s and carefully pipet out the supernatant. DNA will remain bound to the beads during the washing process.
6. Repeat **step 5**.
7. Seal the sample wells on the plate and briefly spin down for 10 s at 1000 rpm to collect the liquid at the bottom of the well.
8. Place the 96-well plate on the magnetic stand for 30 s. Afterward, remove all the remaining ethanol.
9. Place the plate at room temperature for approx. 3–5 min until the pellet appears dry (*see* **Note 3**). You may see a tiny crack in the pellet.
10. Add 12 μL of Purification Buffer to cover the beads. Remove the plate from the magnetic stand and incubate at room temperature for 2 min to rehydrate.
11. Mix the pellet by pipetting up and down 10× to elute DNA from the beads and put the plate back on the magnetic stand until the solution is completely clear (approx. 1 min).
12. Transfer clear supernatant containing purified cDNA from each well to nuclease-free low-retention tubes. For validation using the Agilent 2100 BioAnalyzer and the High Sensitivity DNA Chip from Agilent's High Sensitivity DNA Kit (*see* Subheading 3.5), save a 1 μL aliquot of the amplified cDNA. Store at −20 °C.

3.5 Validation of Purification of ds cDNA Using Agilent 2100 BioAnalyzer

1. Bring the High Sensitivity DNA dye concentrate and High Sensitivity DNA gel matrix to room temperature for approx. 30 min.
2. Vortex the High Sensitivity DNA dye concentrate for 10 s and spin down. Note: Make sure the DMSO is completely thawed.
3. Pipet 15 μL of the High Sensitivity DNA dye concentrate into the vial containing the High Sensitivity DNA gel matrix. The prepared gel–dye mix is sufficient for five chips.
4. Cap the tube, vortex for 10 s, and visually inspect proper mixing of gel and dye.
5. Transfer the complete gel–dye mix to the top receptacle of a spin filter.
6. Place the spin filter in the microcentrifuge and spin for 10 min at room temperature at 2240 *g* ± 20%.
7. Discard the filter according to good laboratory practices. Label the tube and include the date of preparation. Protect from light and store the gel–dye mix at 4 °C when not in use for more than 1 h. Note: Use the gel–dye mix within 6 weeks of preparation.
8. Allow the gel–dye mix to equilibrate to room temperature for approx. 30 min before use while protecting from light.
9. Take a new High Sensitivity DNA chip out of its sealed bag and place the chip on the chip priming station.
10. Pipette 9.0 μL of the gel–dye mix at the bottom of the designated well as per the manufacturer's instructions and dispense the gel–dye mix (*see* **Note 4**).
11. Set the timer to 60 s, make sure that the plunger is positioned at 1 mL with the clip lever at the lowest position and close the chip priming station. The lock of the latch will click only when the Priming Station is closed correctly.
12. Press the plunger of the syringe down until it is held by the clip.
13. Wait for exactly 60 s and then release the plunger with the clip release mechanism.
14. Make sure that the plunger moves back at least to the 0.3 mL mark.
15. Wait for 5 s, then slowly pull back the plunger to the 1 mL position.
16. Open the chip priming station.
17. Pipet 9.0 μL of the gel–dye mix in each of the designated wells as per the manufacturer's instructions.
18. For loading the marker, pipet 5 μL of High Sensitivity DNA marker into the well labeled with a ladder symbol and into each

of the remaining 11 sample wells. Note: Do not leave any wells empty, otherwise the chip will not run properly (*see* **step 20**).

19. For loading the ladder, pipet 1 μL of the High Sensitivity DNA ladder in the well labeled with the ladder symbol.
20. Pipet 1 μL of your sample or, in case of unused wells, 1 μL of marker in the 11 sample wells.
21. Place the chip horizontally in the adapter of the IKA vortex mixer and make sure not to damage the bulge that fixes the chip during vortexing.
22. Vortex for 60 s at 2400 rpm .
23. Open the lid of the Agilent 2100 Bioanalyzer. Make sure that the electrode cartridge is inserted properly and the chip selector is in the appropriate position.
24. Place the chip carefully into the receptacle and close the lid carefully.
25. Start the run and compare the results for your samples & controls (*see* Fig. 1) in order to verify whether your sample is suitable for further processing.

3.6 Covaris Shearing of Full-Length cDNA

1. Turn ON the Covaris system and the main cooler. Add approx. 1.9 L of distilled deionized water (water level should be within ±3 mm of the "FULL" waterline when the transducer is submerged).
2. Close the door and start the control software. Click "ON" for the degassing button, and degas the water bath for 30 min.
3. Add 65 μL of Purification Buffer to the DNA from Subheading 3.4, **step 12**. Transfer 75 μL of the Purification Buffer + DNA mixture into the 100 μL Covaris tube. Put the sample tubes into the appropriate location on the Sample holder.
4. Set up the process configuration panel to 10% duty, intensity 5, burst cycle 200, time 5 min, Frequency Sweeping Mode.
5. Save the file and click return to go back to the main page.
6. Open the tube holder lid and place the tube holder with sample tubes on the transducer positioning system.
7. Close the tube holder lid and click "START" on the main screen to fragment DNA.
8. After shearing is complete, transfer 75 μL of sheared DNA to 1.5 mL tubes.
9. Proceed to library preparation, Subheading 3.7, using the NEBNext® ChIP-Seq Library Prep Master Mix Set for Illumina® Sequencing.

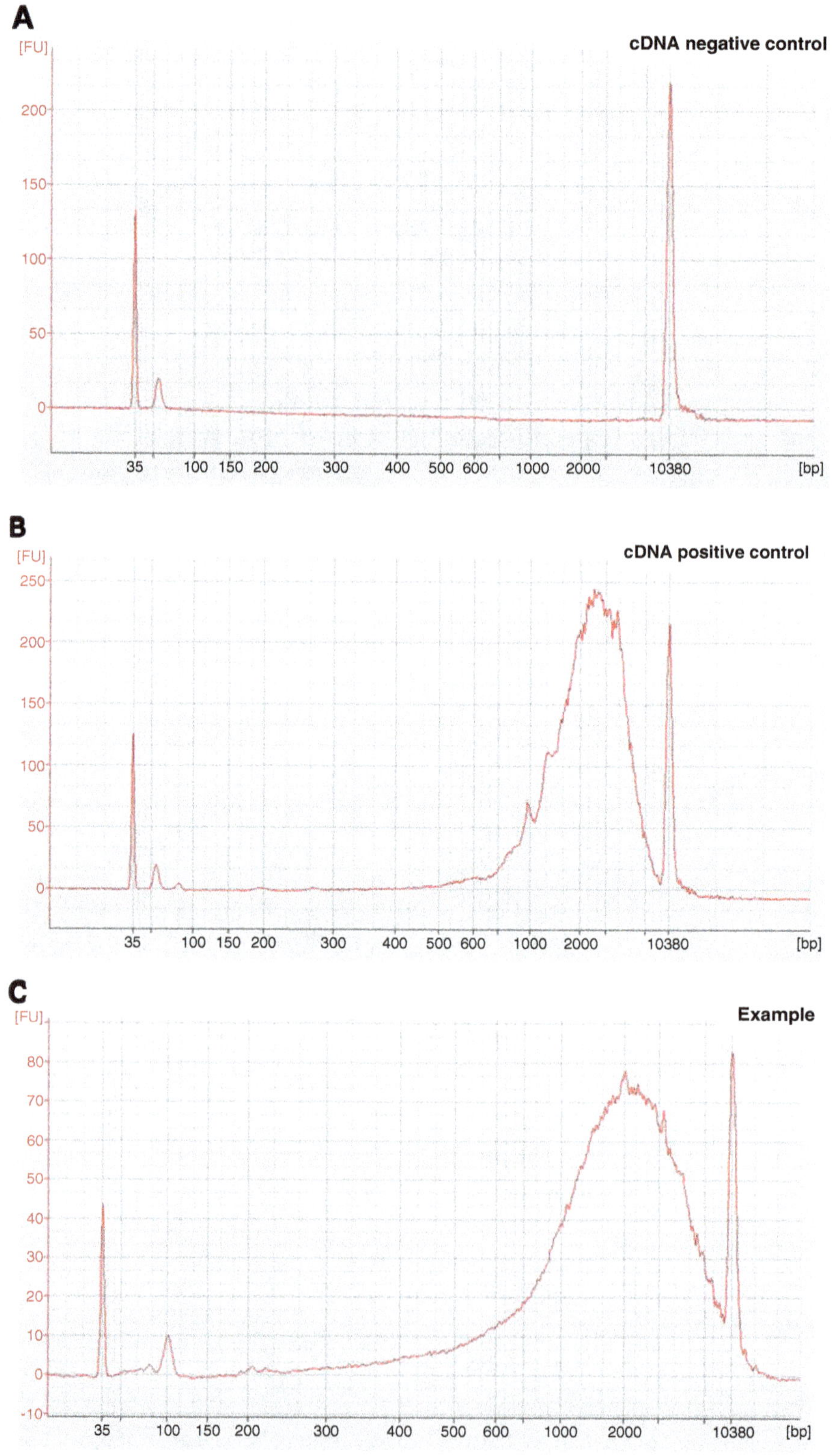

Fig. 1 Validation of cDNA synthesis and amplification using Agilent 2100 BioAnalyzer. In the case of a successful cDNA synthesis and amplification, (**a**) there should be no product in the negative control and (**b**) a distinct peak spanning 400–9000 bp, peaked at approx. 2000 bp for the positive control sample, yielding approximately 2–7 ng of cDNA (depending on the input). (**c**) Contaminated samples have a broader peak and abnormally high cDNA yield

3.7 Library Preparation

1. Mix 10 ng (if less available, take everything) of your fragmented DNA from Subheading 3.6, **step 8**, with 5 μL of NEBNext End Repair Reaction Buffer (10×), and 1 μL of NEBNext End Repair Enzyme Mix. If necessary, add sterile water up to a total volume of 50 μL.
2. Incubate in a thermal cycler for 30 min at 20 °C.
3. For cleanup using AMPure XP® Beads, vortex AMPure XP beads to a homogenous suspension.
4. Add 90 μL (1.8×) of resuspended AMPure XP Beads to the reaction. Mix thoroughly on a vortex mixer or by pipetting up and down at least 10× and incubate for 5 min at room temperature.
5. Place the tube/PCR plate on a magnetic stand to separate beads from supernatant and wait until the solution is clear (approx. 5 min). Carefully remove the supernatant without disturbing the beads containing the DNA fragments. Discard the supernatant.
6. Add 200 μL of 80% freshly prepared ethanol to the tube/PCR plate while on the magnetic stand. Incubate at room temperature for 30 s, and then carefully remove and discard the supernatant.
7. Repeat **step 6**.
8. Air-dry beads for 5 min while the tube/PCR plate is on the magnetic stand with their lids open (*see* **Note 5**).
9. Remove the tube/plate from the magnetic stand and elute the DNA target from the beads by adding 50 μL of 0.1× TE.
10. Mix well on a vortex mixer or by pipetting up and down and incubate for 2 min at room temperature.
11. Put the tube/PCR plate in the magnetic stand until the solution is clear. Carefully transfer 44 μL of the supernatant to a fresh, sterile low retention microfuge tube without disturbing the bead pellet.
12. Mix the following components in a sterile microfuge tube to a total volume of 50 μL: 44 μL of end-repaired/blunt DNA, 5 μL of NEBNext dA-Tailing Reaction Buffer (10×), 1 μL of Klenow Fragment (3′ → 5′ exo-).
13. Incubate in the thermal cycler at 37 °C for 30 min.
14. For cleanup using AMPure XP® Beads, vortex AMPure XP beads to resuspend them.
15. Add 90 μL (1.8×) of resuspended AMPure XP Beads to each reaction. Mix thoroughly on a vortex mixer or by pipetting up and down at least 10× and incubate for 5 min at room temperature.

16. Put the tube/PCR plate on the magnetic stand to separate beads from supernatant and wait until the solution is clear (approx. 5 min). Carefully remove the supernatant without disturbing the beads containing the DNA fragments. Discard the supernatant.
17. Add 200 μL of 80% freshly prepared ethanol to the tube/PCR plate while in the magnetic stand. Incubate at room temperature for 30 s, and then carefully remove and discard the supernatant.
18. Repeat **step 17**.
19. Air-dry beads for 5 min while the tube/PCR plate is on the magnetic stand with the lid open (*see* **Note 5**).
20. Remove the tube/plate from the magnet and elute the DNA target from the beads by adding 25 μL of 0.1× TE.
21. Mix well on a vortex mixer or by pipetting up and down and incubate for 2 min at room temperature.
22. Put the tube/PCR plate in the magnetic stand until the solution is clear. Carefully transfer 19 μL of the supernatant to a fresh, sterile microfuge tube without disturbing the bead pellet. Samples can be stored at −20 °C.
23. Adaptor Ligation of dA-Tailed DNA: dilute the NEBNext Adaptor for Illumina* (15 μM) 10-fold in 10 mM Tris–HCl or 10 mM Tris–HCl with 10 mM NaCl to a final concentration of 1.5 μM.
24. Mix 19 μL of dA-tailed DNA with 6 μL of Quick Ligation Reaction Buffer (5×), 1 μL of diluted NEBNext Adaptor (1.5 μM), and 4 μL of Quick T4 DNA Ligase to a total volume of 30 μL.
25. Incubate in a thermal cycler at 20 °C for 15 min.
26. Add 3 μL of USER™ Enzyme Mix by pipetting up and down, and incubate at 37 °C for 15 min.
27. Cleanup of adaptor ligated DNA, vortex AMPure XP Beads to resuspend them.
28. Add 54 μL of resuspended AMPure XP Beads to the ligation reaction. Mix thoroughly on a vortex mixer or by pipetting up and down at least 10×.
29. Incubate at room temperature for 5 min.
30. Put the tube/PCR plate on a magnetic stand to separate beads from supernatant. Wait until the solution is clear (approx. 5 min), then carefully remove and discard the supernatant without disturbing the beads that contain the DNA targets.
31. Add 200 μL of 80% freshly prepared ethanol to the tube/PCR plate while in the magnetic stand. Incubate at room temperature for 30 s, and then carefully remove and discard the supernatant.

32. Repeat **step 31**.
33. Air-dry beads for 5 min while the tube/PCR plate is on the magnetic stand with the lid open (*see* **Note 5**).
34. Remove the tube/plate from the magnet. Elute the DNA target by adding 105 µL of 10 mM Tris–HCl or 0.1× TE to the beads for bead-based size selection.
35. Mix well on a vortex mixer or by pipetting up and down and incubate for 2 min at room temperature.
36. Put the tube/PCR plate in the magnetic stand until the solution is clear. Transfer 100 µL of supernatant (or desired volume) to a new tube/well, and proceed to bead based size selection.
37. For size selection of DNA with ligated adaptors, add 90 µL (0.9×) of resuspended AMPure XP Beads to 100 µL of DNA solution. Mix well on a vortex mixer or by pipetting up and down at least 10×.
38. Incubate at room temperature for 5 min.
39. Place the tube/PCR plate on a magnetic stand to separate beads from supernatant until the solution is clear (approx. 5 min) and carefully transfer the supernatant to a new tube/well. Discard beads that contain the large fragments.
40. Add 20 µL (0.2×) of resuspended AMPure XP Beads to the supernatant, mix well and incubate at room temperature for 5 min.
41. Put the tube/PCR plate on a magnetic stand to separate beads from supernatant. Wait until the solution is clear (approx. 5 min), carefully remove and discard the supernatant without disturbing the beads that contain DNA targets.
42. Add 200 µL of freshly prepared 80% ethanol to the tube/PCR plate while in the magnetic stand. Incubate at room temperature for 30 s, then carefully remove and discard the supernatant.
43. Repeat **step 42**.
44. Air-dry beads for 5 min while the tube/PCR plate is on the magnetic stand with the lid open.
45. Remove the tube/plate from the magnet and elute the DNA target from the beads by adding 22 µL of 10 mM Tris–HCl or 0.1× TE.
46. Mix well on a vortex mixer or by pipetting up and down and incubate at room temperature for 2 min.
47. Put the tube/PCR plate in the magnetic stand until the solution is clear. Carefully transfer 20 µL of the supernatant to a clean PCR tube without disturbing the bead pellet, and proceed to amplification.

48. For PCR amplification of adaptor-ligated DNA, mix the following components in sterile strip tubes to a total volume of 50 μL: 20 μL of Adaptor-Ligated DNA Fragments, 2.5 μL of Index Primer, 2.5 μL of Universal PCR Primer, and 25 μL of NEBNext Q5 Hot Start HiFi PCR Master Mix (*see* **Note 6**). NEBNext® Multiplex Oligos for Illumina® (Index Primers Set 1) (New England BioLabs, E7335) are included in the Library Prep Kit.
49. Start thermal cycling using the following PCR cycling conditions:

    98 °C 30 s

    15 cycles:

    98 °C 10 s

    65 °C 75 s

    65 °C 5 min

    10 °C ∞

50. For cleanup, vortex AMPure XP Beads to resuspend them.
51. Add 45 μL (0.9×) of resuspended AMPure XP Beads to the PCR reactions (approx. 50 μL). Mix well on a vortex shaker or by pipetting up and down at least 10×.
52. Incubate at room temperature for 5 min.
53. Put the tube/PCR plate on an appropriate magnetic stand to separate beads from supernatant. Wait until the solution is clear (approx. 5 min), then carefully remove and discard the supernatant without disturbing the beads that contain the DNA targets.
54. Add 200 μL of freshly prepared 80% ethanol to the tube/PCR plate while in the magnetic stand. Incubate at room temperature for 30 s, and then carefully remove and discard the supernatant.
55. Repeat **step 54**.
56. Air-dry the beads for 5 min while the tube/PCR plate is on the magnetic stand with the lid open (*see* **Note 5**).
57. Remove the tube/plate from the magnet and elute the DNA target from the beads by adding 30 μL of 0.1× TE.
58. Mix well on a vortex mixer or by pipetting up and down and incubate for 2 min at room temperature.
59. Put the tube/PCR plate in the magnetic stand until the solution is clear. Carefully transfer 25 μL of the supernatant to a clean low-binding microcentrifuge tube without disturbing the bead pellet. Libraries can be stored at −20 °C.
60. Dilute 2–3 μL of the sequencing library 20× with 10 mM Tris–HCl or 0.1× TE and assess the library quality on an Agilent 2100 BioAnalyzer High Sensitivity Chip, *see* Subheading 3.5 and Fig. 2.

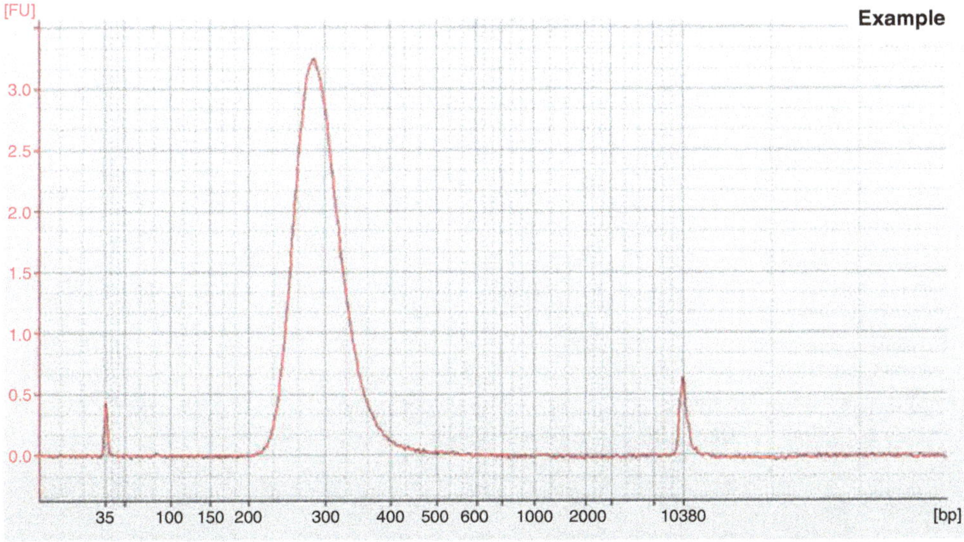

Fig. 2 Bioanalyzer traces of final library. Electropherogram should show a narrow distribution with a peak size of 200–500 bp

3.8 Sequencing

Preparing the reagent cartridge

1. Remove the reagent cartridge from the −25 °C to −15 °C storage.
2. Thaw in a room temperature water bath until thawed (takes approx. 60 min; *see* **Note 7**). Do not submerge the cartridge.
3. Gently tap on the bench to dislodge water from the base, and then dry the base.
4. Invert the cartridge five times to mix reagents.
5. Make sure that reagents are thawed completely and tap gently on the bench to reduce air bubbles.
   Preparing the flow cell
6. Remove a new flow cell package from the 2 °C to 8 °C storage and set the unwrapped flow cell package aside at room temperature for 30 min.
7. Take the flow cell out of the foil package and open the clear plastic clamshell package to remove the flow cell.
8. Clean the glass surface of the flow cell with a lint-free alcohol wipe and dry the glass with a low-lint lab tissue.
   Preparing libraries for sequencing
9. Prepare a fresh dilution of 200 mM NaOH.
10. For preparation of HT1 buffer, remove HT1 from the −25 °C to −15 °C storage and thaw at room temperature.

Table 2
Denature libraries—NaOH

Starting library concentration (nM)	Library (μL)	200 mM NaOH (μL)
4	5	5
2	10	10
1	20	20
0.5	40	40

Table 3
Denature libraries—Tris–HCl

Starting library concentration (nM)	200 mM Tris–HCl[a] (μL)
4	5
2	10
1	20
0.5	40

[a]pH 7

11. Store at 2–8 °C until you are ready to dilute denatured libraries.
Denature libraries
12. Combine equal volumes of library and freshly diluted 200 mM NaOH in the 1.5 mL microcentrifuge tube. *See* Table 2 for relation of library concentration to the required volume.
13. Vortex briefly and then centrifuge at 280 × *g* for 1 min.
14. Incubate at room temperature for 5 min.
15. Add the volume of 200 mM Tris–HCl, pH 7 equal to the initial library volume. *See* Table 3 for guidance.
16. Vortex briefly and then centrifuge at 280 × *g* for 1 min.
17. Dilute denatured libraries to 20 pM solution (*see* Table 4 for guidance).
18. Vortex briefly and then centrifuge at 280 × *g* for 1 min.
19. Place the 20 pM libraries on ice until you are ready to proceed to final dilution.
Dilute libraries to loading concentration
20. Dilute the denatured 20 pM library solution to 1.8 pM solution to a total volume of 1.3 mL: 117 μL denatured library solution +1183 μL prechilled HT1.
21. Invert to mix and then pulse centrifuge. Afterward, store at ice.

Table 4
Denature libraries—HT1

Starting library concentration (nM)	Prechilled HT1 (μL)
4	985
2	970
1	940
0.5	880

Loading Illumina NextSeq®500 System

22. For loading libraries onto the reagent cartridge, clean the foil seal covering reservoir #10 labeled "Load Library Here" using a low-lint tissue.
23. Pierce the seal with a clean 1 mL pipette tip.
24. Load 1.3 mL of prepared 1.8 pM libraries from **step 20** into reservoir #10 labeled "Load Library Here". Avoid touching the foil seal as you dispense the libraries.
    Set up a sequencing run
25. From the Home screen, select Sequence.
26. The Sequence command opens the imaging compartment door, releases consumables from a previous run, and opens the series of run setup screens. A short delay is normal.
27. If the instrument is configured for BaseSpace, you are prompted to log in to BaseSpace.
28. If the instrument is configured for stand-alone mode, the next step is loading the flow cell.
    Load the Flow Cell
29. If necessary, remove the used flow cell from a previous run.
30. Align the flow cell over the alignment pins and place the flow cell on the stage.
31. Select Load.
32. The door closes automatically, the flow cell ID appears on the screen, and the sensors are checked.
33. Select Next.
34. Remove the spent reagents container and discard the contents in accordance with applicable standards.
35. Slide the empty spent reagents container into the buffer compartment until it stops. An audible click indicates that the container is in position.
36. Remove the used buffer cartridge from the upper compartment.

37. Slide a new buffer cartridge into the buffer compartment until it stops.
38. An audible click indicates that the cartridge is in position, the buffer cartridge ID appears on the screen, and the sensor is checked.
39. Close the buffer compartment door, and select Next.
40. If necessary, remove the used reagent cartridge from the reagent compartment.
41. Slide the reagent cartridge into the reagent compartment until the cartridge stops, and then close the reagent compartment door.
42. Select Load.
43. The software moves the cartridge into position automatically (approx. 30 s), the reagent cartridge ID appears on the screen, and the sensors are checked.
44. Select Next.
45. Specify Run Parameters.
46. Enter a run name of your preference.
47. [Optional] Enter a library ID of your preference.
48. From the Recipe drop-down list, select a recipe. Only compatible recipes are listed.
49. Select read type Paired End.
50. Enter the number of cycles for each read in the sequencing run.

    Read 1—Enter a value of 75 cycles.

    Read 2—Enter a value of 75 cycles.

    Index 1—Enter the number of six cycles required for the Index 1 (i7) primer.

    Index 2—Leave the field empty for the Index 2 (i5) primer.
51. Select Next.
52. The software performs an automated check of the system. During the check, the following indicators appear on the screen:

    Gray checkmark—The check has not been performed yet.

    Progress icon—The check is in progress.

    Green checkmark—The check passed.

    Red X—The check did not pass. For any items that do not pass, an action is required before you can proceed.
53. When the automated check is complete, select Start. The sequencing run begins. We suggest to aim for as many as 400 M paired end reads using the High Output Kit.

3.9 First Data Analysis

1. Illumina tool bcl2fastq is used for converting images coming out of the sequencer to fastq files.
2. During this step, sequence reads generated from the pool of individually indexed libraries are deconvoluted according to indices used during library preparation (*see* Subheading 3.7).
3. Quality can be checked on fastqc files by fastQC software: https://www.bioinformatics.babraham.ac.uk/projects/fastqc/.
4. We are using the bwa-mem tool for the alignment to the reference genome:
   http://bio-bwa.sourceforge.net/.
5. Data is now ready for further analysis.

4 Notes

1. Pre-PCR steps such as first-strand cDNA synthesis (Subheading 3.1.) and purification of first-strand cDNA (Subheading 3.2) are suggested to be performed in clean room conditions to avoid contamination of the RNA sample(s). Standard clean room procedures should be followed.
2. Delays after **step 4** of the First-Strand cDNA Synthesis should be avoided. The initial reaction steps (**steps 5–7**) are critical for the first-strand synthesis and should not be delayed after the **step 4**. You can prepare your master mix (for **step 5**) while your tubes are incubating (**step 4**) in order to jump-start the cDNA synthesis.
3. In case of beads were overdried during purification of ds cDNA, many cracks in the pellet will be visible. If it is underdried, the DNA recovery rate will be lower because of the remaining ethanol.
4. When pipetting the gel–dye mix, make sure not to draw up particles that may sit at the bottom of the vial. Insert the tip of the pipette to the bottom of the chip-well when dispensing instead of placing the pipette at the edge of the well to avoid poor results. This prevents a large air bubble forming under the gel–dye mix.
5. Do not overdry the beads during library preparation as this may result in lower recovery of DNA fragments.
6. A precipitate can form upon thawing of the NEBNext Q5 Hot Start HiFi PCR Master Mix. Place the master mix at room temperature while performing cleanup of adaptor-ligated DNA to ensure optimal performance. Once thawed, gently mix by inverting the tube several times.
7. Reagent cartridge: Reagents can also be thawed overnight at 2–8 °C (requires a minimum of 18 h). At this temperature, reagents are stable up to 1 week.

Acknowledgments

This work was in part supported by grants from the German Federal Ministry of Education (BMBF) within the framework of the e:Med research and funding concept "CLIOMMICS" (01ZX1309 and 01ZX1609) and the Deutsche Forschungsgemeinschaft (DFG SFB/TRR79; TP B1 and B12).

References

1. Neben K, Jauch A, Hielscher T, Hillengass J, Lehners N, Seckinger A, Granzow M, Raab MS, Ho AD, Goldschmidt H, Hose D (2013) Progression in smoldering myeloma is independently determined by the chromosomal abnormalities del(17p), t(4;14), gain 1q, hyperdiploidy, and tumor load. J Clin Oncol 31(34):4325–4332
2. Seckinger A, Hose D (2015) Dissecting the Clonal Architecture of Multiple Myeloma. Paper presented at the 20th Congress of the European Hematology Association, Vienna, Austria
3. Hose D, Moreaux J, Meissner T, Seckinger A, Goldschmidt H, Benner A, Mahtouk K, Hillengass J, Rème T, Vos JD, Hundemer M, Condomines M, Bertsch U, Rossi J-F, Jauch A, Klein B, Möhler T (2009) Induction of angiogenesis by normal and malignant plasma cells. Blood 114(1):128–143
4. Hose D, Reme T, Hielscher T, Moreaux J, Meissner T, Seckinger A, Benner A, Shaughnessy JD, Barlogie B, Zhou Y, Hillengass J, Bertsch U, Neben K, Mohler T, Rossi JF, Jauch A, Klein B, Goldschmidt H (2011) Proliferation is a central independent prognostic factor and target for personalized and risk adapted treatment in multiple myeloma. Haematologica 96:87–95
5. Hose D, Rème T, Meissner T, Moreaux J, Seckinger A, Lewis J, Benes V, Benner A, Hundemer M, Hielscher T, Shaughnessy JD, Barlogie B, Neben K, Krämer A, Hillengass J, Bertsch U, Jauch A, Vos JD, Rossi J-F, Möhler T, Blake J, Zimmermann J, Klein B, Goldschmidt H (2009) Inhibition of aurora kinases for tailored risk-adapted treatment of multiple myeloma. Blood 113(18):4331–4340
6. Seckinger A, Meißner T, Moreaux J, Depeweg D, Hillengass J, Hose K, Reme T, Rosen-Wolff A, Jauch A, Schnettler R, Ewerbeck V, Goldschmidt H, Klein B, Hose D (2012) Clinical and prognostic role of annexin A2 in multiple myeloma. Blood 120(5):1087–1094. https://doi.org/10.1182/blood-2012-03-415588
7. Seckinger A, Meissner T, Moreaux J, Goldschmidt H, Fuhler GM, Benner A, Hundemer M, Rème T, Shaughnessy JD, Barlogie B, Bertsch U, Hillengass J, Ho AD, Pantesco V, Jauch A, Vos JD, Rossi JF, Möhler T, Klein B, Hose D (2009) Bone morphogenic protein 6: a member of a novel class of prognostic factors expressed by normal and malignant plasma cells inhibiting proliferation and angiogenesis. Oncogene 28(44):3866–3879
8. Avet-Loiseau H, Attal M, Moreau P, Charbonnel C, Garban F, Hulin C, Leyvraz S, Michallet M, Yakoub-Agha I, Garderet L, Marit G, Michaux L, Voillat L, Renaud M, Grosbois B, Guillerm G, Benboubker L, Monconduit M, Thieblemont C, Casassus P, Caillot D, Stoppa A-M, Sotto J-J, Wetterwald M, Dumontet C, Fuzibet J-G, Azais I, Dorvaux V, Zandecki M, Bataille R, Minvielle S, Harousseau J-L, Facon T, Mathiot C (2007) Genetic abnormalities and survival in multiple myeloma: the experience of the Intergroupe francophone du Myelome. Blood 109(8): 3489–3495
9. Meißner T, Seckinger A, Rème T, Hielscher T, Möhler T, Neben K, Goldschmidt H, Klein B, Hose D (2011) Gene expression profiling in multiple myeloma--reporting of entities, risk, and targets in clinical routine. Clin Cancer Res 17(23):7240–7247
10. Shaughnessy JD, Zhan F, Burington BE, Huang Y, Colla S, Hanamura I, Stewart JP, Kordsmeier B, Randolph C, Williams DR, Xiao Y, Xu H, Epstein J, Anaissie E, Krishna SG, Cottler-Fox M, Hollmig K, Mohiuddin A, Pineda-Roman M, Tricot G, van Rhee F, Sawyer J, Alsayed Y, Walker R, Zangari M, Crowley J, Barlogie B (2007) A validated gene expression model of high-risk multiple myeloma is defined by deregulated expression of genes mapping to chromosome 1. Blood 109(6):2276–2284

11. Reme T, Hose D, Theillet C, Klein B (2013) Modeling risk stratification in human cancer. Bioinformatics 29(9):1149–1157. https://doi.org/10.1093/bioinformatics/btt124
12. Decaux O, Lodé L, Magrangeas F, Charbonnel C, Gouraud W, Jézéquel P, Attal M, Harousseau J-L, Moreau P, Bataille R, Campion L, Avet-Loiseau H, Minvielle S, du Myélome IF (2008) Prediction of survival in multiple myeloma based on gene expression profiles reveals cell cycle and chromosomal instability signatures in high-risk patients and hyperdiploid signatures in low-risk patients: a study of the Intergroupe francophone du Myélome. J Clin Oncol 26(29):4798–4805
13. Bergsagel PL, Kuehl WM, Zhan F, Sawyer J, Barlogie B, Shaughnessy J (2005) Cyclin D dysregulation: an early and unifying pathogenic event in multiple myeloma. Blood 106(1):296–303
14. Zhan F, Huang Y, Colla S, Stewart JP, Hanamura I, Gupta S, Epstein J, Yaccoby S, Sawyer J, Burington B, Anaissie E, Hollmig K, Pineda-Roman M, Tricot G, van Rhee F, Walker R, Zangari M, Crowley J, Barlogie B, Shaughnessy JD (2006) The molecular classification of multiple myeloma. Blood 108(6):2020–2028
15. Seckinger A, Delgado JA, Moser S, Moreno L, Neuber B, Grab A, Lipp S, Merino J, Prosper F, Emde M, Delon C, Latzko M, Gianotti R, Lüoend R, Murr R, Hosse RJ, Harnisch LJ, Bacac M, Fauti T, Klein C, Zabaleta A, Hillengass J, Cavalcanti-Adam EA, Ho AD, Hundemer M, San Miguel JF, Strein K, Umaña P, Hose D, Paiva B, Vu MD (2017) Target expression, generation, preclinical activity, and pharmacokinetics of the BCMA-T cell bispecific antibody EM801 for multiple myeloma treatment. Cancer Cell 31(3):396–410
16. Andrulis M, Lehners N, Capper D, Penzel R, Heining C, Huellein J, Zenz T, von Deimling A, Schirmacher P, Ho AD, Goldschmidt H, Neben K, Raab MS (2013) Targeting the BRAF V600E mutation in multiple myeloma. Cancer Discov 3(8):862–869. https://doi.org/10.1158/2159-8290.CD-13-0014
17. Seckinger A, Meissner T, Moreaux J, Benes V, Hillengass J, Castoldi M, Zimmermann J, Ho AD, Jauch A, Goldschmidt H, Klein B, Hose D (2015) miRNAs in multiple myeloma—a survival relevant complex regulator of gene expression. Oncotarget 6(36):39165–39183. https://doi.org/10.18632/oncotarget.5381

Chapter 8

Protocol for M³P: A Comprehensive and Clinical Oriented Targeted Sequencing Panel for Routine Molecular Analysis in Multiple Myeloma

Santiago Barrio, Matteo DáVia, Laura Bruins, Thorsten Stühmer, Torsten Steinbrunn, Max Bittrich, Hermann Einsele, Alexander Keith Stewart, Esteban Braggio, and Klaus Martin Kortüm

Abstract

Over the past 10 years next generation sequencing (NGS) approaches deciphered a large number of genomes from a wide variety of tumor types. However, despite most relevant findings, this technology has not yet been implemented into standard diagnostic workflows. Broad access to NGS technology is still limited, sequencing/analysis times exceed clinically relevant timeframes and despite huge cuts, costs remain significant. We proposed a custom-tailored gene panel, which focuses on a selected number of relevant genes and developed a clinically oriented NGS targeted sequencing approach for the molecular characterization of Multiple Myeloma (MM) tumors, allowing the description of the tumor genetic heterogeneity and its changes under selective pressure of antitumor therapy, in a more cost effective and faster turnaround timeframe.

Key words Multiple myeloma, Next generation sequencing, Targeted sequencing panel, Standard diagnostic workflow

1 Introduction

Since its discovery, DNA sequencing has impacted research and our understanding of cancer significantly. The arrival of massively parallel next generation sequencing methodologies allow the rapid generation of large amounts of genetic information and to date the molecular landscape of most tumors has been described. This includes multiple myeloma (MM), which is the second most common hematologic malignancy and the main focus of our group [1–4]. Available MM genomic data mainly restrict on untreated disease and data from whole genome/exome sequencing analyses (WGS and WES). We and others have suggested that the subclonal composition of MM tumors are of importance for the better

Christoph Heuck and Niels Weinhold (eds.), *Multiple Myeloma: Methods and Protocols*, Methods in Molecular Biology, vol. 1792, https://doi.org/10.1007/978-1-4939-7865-6_8,

understanding for disease evolvement under the selective pressures of therapy and the development of drug resistance [5–7].

Target deep sequencing (TDS) leverages from the available genomic information and allows a more detailed mutational picture of selected genes. In some cases it seems to be sufficient to focus on specific coding regions within genes of interest, e.g., in the case of a known "hotspot" mutation. Variable software tools can be used to visualize the data obtained, including open access platforms like the Integrative Genome Viewer (IGV) [8] with which gene sequences can be visualized and compared to a reference human genome [9, 10].

TDS may be used to facilitate the transfer genomic information 'from the bench to the bedside', here it benefits from more economic and faster result availability, compared to more comprehensive genome sequencing and results are highly sensitive, specific and reproducible [6, 11]. We developed a MM-specific mutation panel (M^3P). In its current version (v3.0), it includes a selection of 88 genes that represent genes known to be either recurrently mutated in MM, that are critical pathway components, that are related to drug resistance against the most commonly used MM therapies (steroids, proteasome inhibitors and immunomodulators) or provide actionable targets for individualized treatment strategies. The M^3P has been successfully validated analyzing more than 500 MM cases so far [5, 12–15]. We identified mutations in 83% of the patients demonstrating that the M^3P panel covers the genetic landscape of MM. In most of the genes we found an increased rate of mutations, notably, this includes a significant number of mutations within low frequency clones that would have been undetectable by standard resolution WES. In this chapter we describe the protocol now in use for the molecular characterization of multiple myeloma samples and how the derived information could be translated to the clinic (*see* **Note 1**).

2 Materials

2.1 DNA Isolation

1. Kit of election.
2. 70% ethanol.

2.2 Library Preparation

1. Ion AmpliSeq Library Kit 2.0 (Life Technologies).
2. IonXpress Barcode Adapters 1-16 Kit (Life Technologies).
3. Nuclease-free water.
4. PCR machine.
5. Vortex.
6. Mini centrifuge.
7. PCR tube strip.

2.3 Library Purification

1. AMPure Beads: AMPure XP (Beckman Coulter).
2. 70% ethanol.
3. DynaMag™-96 Side Magnet (Thermo).
4. Low TE Buffer.
5. Lo-Bind tubes.

2.4 Quantification of Library Products with qPCR

1. Ion Library TaqMan Quantitation Kit (Life Technologies).
2. Nuclease-free water.
3. MicroAmp Fast 96-well Reaction Plate, 0.1 mL (Life Technologies).
4. Self-adhesive film (Applied Biosystems).
5. qPCR machine (StepOne plus or equivalent machine).

2.5 Emulsion PCR

1. Ion PGM Hi-Q OT2 Reagents (Life Technologies).
2. Reaction oil.
3. 1 M NaOH solution (appr. 1 mL).
4. Ion OneTouch 2.

2.6 Washing ISPs

1. Kit: Ion PGM Hi-Q OT2 Reagents (Life Technologies).
2. 1 M NaOH solution.
3. Beads- Ion PGM enrichment beads (Life Technologies).
4. Ion OneTouch ES.

2.7 Quantification of ISPs

1. Annealing Buffer.
2. Ion Sphere Quality Control Kit (Life Technologies).
3. Wash Buffer.
4. Qubit tubes.
5. Centrifuge.
6. PCR machine.

2.8 Sequencing

1. 100 mM NaOH solution.
2. ION PGM HI-Q SEQ KIT (Life Technologies).
3. LoBind tubes.
4. PGM Sequencer.

3 Methods

3.1 DNA Isolation (See Note 2)

We applied our panel to different sources of MM cells (paraffin embedded biopsies, liquid biopsies and bone marrow cells) and we were able to detect somatic mutations in as low as 10 cells (unpublished data). However, we highly recommend to use CD138 cells purified from bone marrow aspirates (by sorting on magnetic beads). Samples from CRs or samples diluted during the aspiration extraction may have low number of purified cells. We have defined an internal threshold of 10,000 plasma cells as the minimum quantity for routine diagnosis. The DNA isolation method can be selected by the user, we recommend to use an ethanol precipitation approach, of which we experienced a high yield of good quality DNA with Puregene kit (Qiagen).

3.2 Library Preparation (See Note 3)

1. For each sample label two PCR tubes designated for primer pool 1 and primer pool 2, respectively.
2. Add 2 μL of 5× Ion AmpliSeq HiFi Mix (red cap) to each tube (*see* **Note 4**).
3. For primer pool 1 or 2 respectively add 5 μL to the appropriate tubes.
4. Add 10 ng of DNA sample to appropriate tubes and add nuclease-free water to a final volume of 10 μL. Ensure that the amount of DNA is the same for pool 1 or 2 respectively.
5. Mix the samples by tapping with your finger, give a short spin and place tubes in the PCR cycler. We recommend using one extra cycle than what is listed by Thermo fisher. For M^{3}P panel we use 17 cycles.

   1-Amplification PCR program:

   Stage 1: 99 °C, 2 min

   Stage 2: 2 cycles

   99 °C, 15 s

   62 °C, 4 min

   Stage 3: 15 cycles

   99 °C, 15 s

   60 °C, 4 min

   Hold 10 °C

   After this step products may be stored at −20 °C.

6. Spin down to recover all the content of the tube and combine primer pools of each sample into one of the tubes. Once combined add 2 μL of FuPa Reagent (brown cap) to all tubes, mix and spin down briefly. Using the PCR cycler again, run the following program:

   2-Digestion program:

   50 °C for 20 min

   55 °C for 20 min

60 °C for 20 min

Hold at 10 °C (up to 1 h)

7. During the digestion program prepare the barcodes mixes: Dilute 2 µL of each barcode with 2 µL of adapter and 4 µL of nuclease-free water. Diluted barcodes may be stored at −20 °C.
8. Continue immediately after the second PCR step and add 4 µL of Switch Solution (yellow cap) to all samples. Add 2 µL of appropriate barcode to the tubes and avoid any cross contamination. Finally, add 2 µL of Ligase (blue cap) to all tubes, mix, give a short spin and run following program in the PCR cycler:

   3-Ligation Program:

   22 °C for 30 min

   68 °C for 5 min

   72 °C for 5 min

   Hold at 10 °C (up to 24 h)
   The products may be stored at −20 °C.

3.3 Purify the Library

1. Label new tubes for final purified product. Keep aside.
2. Bring beads and samples to room temperature and prepare 70% ethanol (appr. 10 mL).
3. Vortex the beads for 1 min and add 45 µL to each sample. Mix properly by pipetting up and down and incubate at room temperature for 5 min.
4. Place the tubes in a magnetic rack for 2 min, and then carefully discard the supernatant.
5. Wash each tube with 150 µL of 70% ethanol (using a multichannel pipet). By changing the tubes from one side of the magnetic rack to the other 4–6 times the beads are washed properly. Keep tube on rack for 2 min.
6. Discard supernatant and perform a second wash step as described above.
7. Subsequently, remove ethanol without any residual drops then let it air-dry for 5 min.
8. Get the tubes off the magnetic rack and add 50 µL of low TE Buffer. Mix with a pipet, give the tubes a short spin and put back into the magnetic rack for another 2 min.
9. Carefully transfer the supernatant which contains the purified DNA into the new tubes and store at −20 °C.

3.4 Quantification of Library Products with qPCR

1. Different sample dilutions are required for the assay. For each sample a 1:200 and a 1:2000 dilution should be run in duplicates. First prepare a 1:20 dilution with nuclease-free water and from that make the two other dilutions required (Table 1).

Table 1
Sample dilutions for library qPCR

	DNA (μL)	Water (μL)
1:20	4	76
1:200	4 of 1:20	36
1:2000	4 of 1:200	36

Table 2
Standards dilutions

	Std DNA (μL)	Water (μL)
Std 1	5	0
Std 2	5	45
Std 3	5 of Std 2	45
Std 4	5 of Std 3	45
Std 5	5 of Std 4	45
Std 6	5 of Std 5	45
Std 7	5 of Std 6	45
Blank	0	45

2. Close the tubes with recommended lids while leaving at room temperature.
3. Prepare standard (yellow cap) dilutions as seen in Table 2 (*see* **Note 5**).
4. Prepare a qPCR plate and add 15 μL of water to all wells of columns 1 and 12 and all unused wells.
5. To all wells designated for standards or samples add 5 μL of Ion Library TaqMan qPCR Master Mix, 2× (blue cap), 0.5 μL of Ion Library TaqMan Quantitation Assay, 20× (red cap) and 2 μL of water or prepare a master mix of the three reagents and add 7.5 μL of it to each well.
6. Add 2.5 μL of each standard or sample to the appropriate wells and mix by gently pipetting up and down. Standards and all samples should be run in duplicates.
7. Seal the plate with a self-adhesive film and ensure that the film covers the plate everywhere to avoid evaporation.
8. Before starting the qPCR run give the plate a short spin.

3.5 Emulsion PCR

1. By diluting with low TE buffer adjust the samples to a concentration of 100 pM.
2. Prepare a library pool by adding 10 μL of each diluted sample to a fresh 1.5 mL tube.
3. Dilute the library pool again by mixing 3 μL of it with 22 μL of water in another tube.
4. Bring Ion PGM Hi-Q ISPs and Ion PGM Hi-Q Reagent Mix to room temperature and keep Ion PGM Hi-Q Enzyme Mix on ice.
5. Start with the cleaning procedure and the instrument setup of the Ion OneTouch by following the instructions of the machine. Add appropriate volumes of oil and recovery solutions to designated bottles. Insert new plate, centrifuge tubes and routers.
6. Add 150 μL breaking solution to each tube. Close centrifuge lid and insert needle into position.
7. Vortex the Ion PGM Hi-Q Reagent Mix (brown cap) and the Ion PGM Hi-Q ISPs (black cap) properly.
8. Add all reagents required directly into the tube of the Ion PGM Hi-Q Reagent Mix (purple tube): 25 μL of Nuclease-free water, 50 μL of Ion PGM Hi-Q Enzyme Mix, 25 μL of diluted library pool, and 100 μL of Ion PGM Hi-Q ISPs. The latter should be vortexed again prior to use.
9. Vortex the amplification solution for 5 s and bear in mind that the solution is stable for only 15 min.
10. Apply the complete amplification solution (final volume 1 mL) to a new reaction filter, avoid bubbles and with a 1000 μL pipet carefully add two times 850 μL of Reaction oil to overlay the solution.
11. Turn over the reaction filter as described in the protocol, insert into the machine and start the run.
12. After finishing the run perform a final centrifugation step.
13. Take out the recovery tubes, remove the supernatant except 50 μL (if desired see comparatively tube), resuspend both pellets in the residual liquid and transfer the content of both tubes into a fresh 1.5 mL LoBind tube.
14. Wash recovery tubes again with 500 μL of Ion OneTouch Wash Solution and add everything to the LoBind tube. This product may be stored at 4 °C for 3 days.
15. Centrifuge for 2.5 min at 15,500 × *g*, discard supernatant except 100 μL and resuspend the pellet in residual liquid.
16. Take aside approximately 2 μL of the ISPs into a new 0.2-mL tube for the ISPs quantification.

17. Continue with the ISPs quantification and start with the cleaning of the Ion OneTouch 2 machine.

3.6 Washing ISPs

1. Prepare 8well strip (square end of the strip to the left, round to the right) and transfer the complete ISPs sample from **step 5** into well 1.
2. Prepare Melt-off solution by mixing 40 μL of 1 M NaOH and 280 μL of Tween Solution in a 1.5-mL tube and transfer 300 μL in well 7 of the 8well strip.
3. Vortex Ion PGM Enrichment Beads and add 13 μL to a LoBind tube.
4. Put on a magnet and leave for 2 min before removing the supernatant.
5. Add 130 μL of Beads Wash Solution, vortex, give a short spin and transfer in well 2 of the 8well strip.
6. Add 30 μL of Ion OneTouch Wash Solution into wells 3, 4 and 5.
7. Place the 8well strip at the Ion OneTouch ES machine, ensure the right alignment of the strip and continue with the machine setup.
8. Attach a new pipet tip to the adapter and place a new PCR tube with 10 μL of Neutralization Solution in the designated hole.

3.7 Quantification of ISPs

1. Add 19 μL of Annealing Buffer to the 2 μL of ISPs (*see* Subheading 3.5, **step 13**).
2. Add 1 μL of Ion Sphere Quality Control Kit Ion Probes, mix and incubate in a thermal cycler for 2 min at 95 °C and another 2 min at 37 °C.
3. Wash three times with 200 μL wash buffer, each time centrifuge at 15,000 × *g* for 2 min and take out supernatant except ~15 μL.
4. Resuspend the 15 μL in a final volume of 200 μL of Wash Buffer and transfer to a Qubit tube.
5. Use Wash Buffer as a blank control. Measure absorbance of the ISPs at 488 nm and 647 nm respectively. The ISPs should be template-positive around 10–30%.

3.8 Sequencing

We do not introduce any modification to the standard PGM sequencing protocol provided by Thermo fisher for 400 bp (850 flows). However, we modify the default variant caller configuration to be sure that we are obtaining all small somatic subclonal mutations (*see* **Note 6**).

3.9 Data Analysis

1. Variant caller files (VCF), BAM files, and BAM.bai files are obtained from the torrent suit.

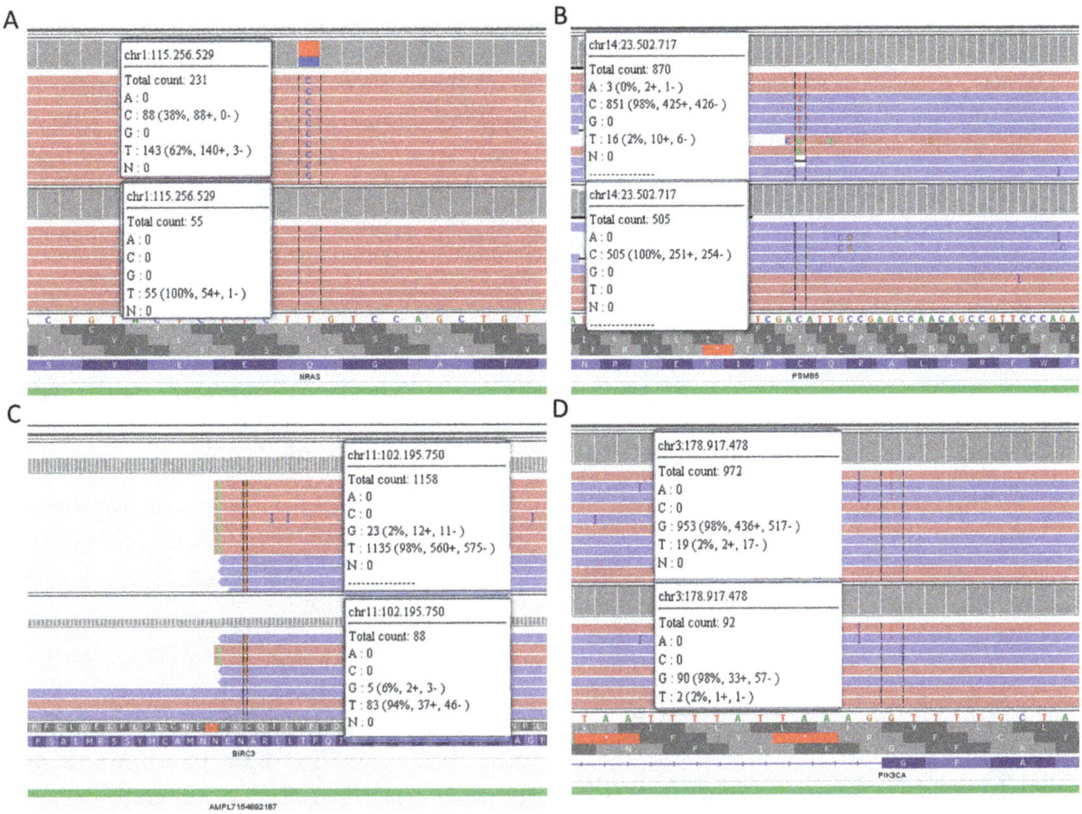

Fig. 1 Examples of different variants. (**a**) Clonal somatic mutations, (**b**) subclonal somatic mutation, (**c**) alignment artifact, and (**d**) homopolymer artifact. Top track in each panel: Tumor sample (CD138 purified cells from a MM case). Bottom: Germ Line (PBMCs cells). Green Line: Region covered by the amplicon. Salmon lines: Forward reads. Blue lines: Reverse reads. Boxes: Total read and variant counts for the selected position

2. VCF files are uploaded to Ion Reporter Software v5.2, and annotated using the "annotate variants single sample workflow".
3. Variants are filtered by a soft filtering chain (*see* **Note** 7). These filters, by only eliminating variants with low VR or low coverage as well as synonymous alterations, allow us to reduce the number of candidates in more than 90% (usually we obtain 250–300 variants that get reduced to 20–40 after filtering).
4. The remaining variants are then further filtered: all variants listed in dbSNP without being listed in the COSMIC database are excluded from further analysis.
5. The remaining findings are further compared with an in-house common error database and then visually screened with the Integrative Genomics Viewer (IGV). This visual inspection allows identifying variants that, despite low allele frequency and coverage, are not artifacts produced by a homopolymer or a poor alignment (Fig. 1) but are noteworthy candidates for validation.

3.10 Validation of Candidates

Validation of candidates is mandatory in all cases by an independent sequencing run using sufficient coverage. Germ line samples are run to distinguish polymorphisms and somatic mutations. Clonal mutations as well as subclonal ones with more than 20% VR can be validated by Sanger sequencing. Low frequency subclonal mutations are validated by NGS using custom primers and the custom library preparation kit (e.g., Thermo Fisher).

4 Notes

1. The present methodology reflects the approach used in the research lab. This is not the methodology and standards the Mayo Clinic clinical lab is using for patient molecular screening.
2. There are many approaches for successful DNA isolation. TDS requires comparably small amounts of starting material which enables to investigate low cell number samples. We recommend an alcoholic DNA precipitation kit, e.g., the Puregene kit (Qiagen). Instead of column approaches, it guarantees the extraction of the entire DNA fraction, independently of the size of the molecules. Also it permits to reduce the elution volumes to increase DNA concentration without reducing DNA yields. In case that the RNA fraction is required, the Micro RNA/DNA kit may be used. However, we only recommend this approach for samples with more than 100,000 cells.
3. In our hands a two-fold reduction of the volumes recommended by Thermo fisher was possible. After the amplification PCR with the Panel pools, we suggest to combine both pools and continue with the protocol as indicated by Thermo Fisher. This allows a more efficient use of reagents, without significantly compromising the uniformity of the reads (around 80–90%).
4. It is possible to use a four-fold library reduction modification, working with four times less reagents in the amplification step, mixing the pools for a final volume of 10 μL and continue with half of volumes for the digestion and ligation. However this approach implies work with low DNA cell equivalents (5 ng, less than 1000 cells equivalents) and an amplification PCR volume of 5 μL.
5. Prepare all solutions using ultrapure water and analytical grade reagents. Diligently follow all waste disposal regulations.
6. Variant caller custom configuration is adjusted to include all possible variants with allele frequency $\leq 1\%$ and coverage ≤ 2 in both strands.
7. Ion reporter filtering chain: $0.01 \leq$ Allele Ratio ≤ 1.0; $4 \leq$ Allele Read-Count $\leq 100{,}000$; Variant Effect; $\neq$ refAllele, $\neq$ synonymous

References

1. Bolli N, Avet-Loiseau H, Wedge DC, Van Loo P, Alexandrov LB, Martincorena I, Dawson KJ, Iorio F, Nik-Zainal S, Bignell GR, Hinton JW, Li Y, Tubio JM, McLaren S, OM S, Butler AP, Teague JW, Mudie L, Anderson E, Rashid N, Tai YT, Shammas MA, Sperling AS, Fulciniti M, Richardson PG, Parmigiani G, Magrangeas F, Minvielle S, Moreau P, Attal M, Facon T, Futreal PA, Anderson KC, Campbell PJ, Munshi NC (2014) Heterogeneity of genomic evolution and mutational profiles in multiple myeloma. Nat Commun 5:2997. https://doi.org/10.1038/ncomms3997
2. Cancer Genome Atlas Research N (2013) Genomic and epigenomic landscapes of adult de novo acute myeloid leukemia. N Engl J Med 368(22):2059–2074. https://doi.org/10.1056/NEJMoa1301689
3. Lohr JG, Stojanov P, Carter SL, Cruz-Gordillo P, Lawrence MS, Auclair D, Sougnez C, Knoechel B, Gould J, Saksena G, Cibulskis K, McKenna A, Chapman MA, Straussman R, Levy J, Perkins LM, Keats JJ, Schumacher SE, Rosenberg M, Multiple Myeloma Research C, Getz G, Golub TR (2014) Widespread genetic heterogeneity in multiple myeloma: implications for targeted therapy. Cancer Cell 25(1):91–101. https://doi.org/10.1016/j.ccr.2013.12.015
4. Walker BA, Boyle EM, Wardell CP, Murison A, Begum DB, Dahir NM, Proszek PZ, Johnson DC, Kaiser MF, Melchor L, Aronson LI, Scales M, Pawlyn C, Mirabella F, Jones JR, Brioli A, Mikulasova A, Cairns DA, Gregory WM, Quartilho A, Drayson MT, Russell N, Cook G, Jackson GH, Leleu X, Davies FE, Morgan GJ (2015) Mutational spectrum, copy number changes, and outcome: results of a sequencing study of patients with newly diagnosed myeloma. J Clin Oncol 33(33):3911–3920. https://doi.org/10.1200/JCO.2014.59.1503
5. Kortuem KM, Braggio E, Bruins L, Barrio S, Shi CS, Zhu YX, Tibes R, Viswanatha D, Votruba P, Ahmann G, Fonseca R, Jedlowski P, Schlam I, Kumar S, Bergsagel PL, Stewart AK (2016) Panel sequencing for clinically oriented variant screening and copy number detection in 142 untreated multiple myeloma patients. Blood Cancer J 6:e397. https://doi.org/10.1038/bcj.2016.1
6. Kortum KM, Mai EK, Hanafiah NH, Shi CX, Zhu YX, Bruins L, Barrio S, Jedlowski P, Merz M, Xu J, Stewart RA, Andrulis M, Jauch A, Hillengass J, Goldschmidt H, Bergsagel PL, Braggio E, Stewart AK, Raab MS (2016) Targeted sequencing of refractory myeloma reveals a high incidence of mutations in CRBN and Ras pathway genes. Blood 128(9):1226–1233. https://doi.org/10.1182/blood-2016-02-698092
7. Kortum KM, Zhu YX, Shi CX, Jedlowski P, Stewart AK (2015) Cereblon binding molecules in multiple myeloma. Blood Rev 29(5):329–334. https://doi.org/10.1016/j.blre.2015.03.003
8. Robinson JT, Thorvaldsdottir H, Winckler W, Guttman M, Lander ES, Getz G, Mesirov JP (2011) Integrative genomics viewer. Nat Biotechnol 29(1):24–26. https://doi.org/10.1038/nbt.1754
9. Okou DT, Steinberg KM, Middle C, Cutler DJ, Albert TJ, Zwick ME (2007) Microarray-based genomic selection for high-throughput resequencing. Nat Methods 4(11):907–909. https://doi.org/10.1038/nmeth1109
10. Shendure J, Ji H (2008) Next-generation DNA sequencing. Nat Biotechnol 26(10):1135–1145. https://doi.org/10.1038/nbt1486
11. Barrio S, Shanafelt TD, Ojha J, Chaffee KG, Secreto C, Kortum KM, Pathangey S, Van-Dyke DL, Slager SL, Fonseca R, Kay NE, Braggio E (2017) Genomic characterization of high-count MBL cases indicates that early detection of driver mutations and subclonal expansion are predictors of adverse clinical outcome. Leukemia 31(1):170–176. https://doi.org/10.1038/leu.2016.172
12. Kortum KM, Langer C, Monge J, Bruins L, Zhu YX, Shi CX, Jedlowski P, Egan JB, Ojha J, Bullinger L, Kull M, Ahmann G, Rasche L, Knop S, Fonseca R, Einsele H, Stewart AK, Braggio E (2015) Longitudinal analysis of 25 sequential sample-pairs using a custom multiple myeloma mutation sequencing panel (MP). Ann Hematol 94(7):1205–1211. https://doi.org/10.1007/s00277-015-2344-9
13. Kortum KM, Langer C, Monge J, Bruins L, Egan JB, Zhu YX, Shi CX, Jedlowski P, Schmidt J, Ojha J, Bullinger L, Liebisch P, Kull M, Champion MD, Van Wier S, Ahmann G, Rasche L, Knop S, Fonseca R, Einsele H, Stewart AK, Braggio E (2015) Targeted sequencing using a 47 gene multiple myeloma mutation panel (M(3) P) in -17p high risk disease. Br J Haematol 168(4):507–510. https://doi.org/10.1111/bjh.13171
14. Kortuem KM, Stewart AK, Bruins LA, Ahmann G, Vasmatzis G, Rajkumar SV, Kumar S, Dispenzieri A, Lacy MQ, Gertz MA, Fonseca R, Champion M, Bergsagel PL, Braggio E (2014) Development and results of a multiple

myeloma specific custom 77-gene mutation panel for clinical targeted sequencing. Blood 124:169

15. Kortüm KM, Braggio E, Sonneveld P, Bruins L, Barrio S, Hofste BD, van Duin M, Mai EK, Hanafiah N, Goldschmidt H, Knop S, Rasche L, Langer C, Kull M, LB, Engelhardt M, Martinez-Lopez J, Einsele H, Raab MS, Stewart AK (2015) Overview of 500 Multiple Myeloma (MM) patients analyzed by targeted sequencing at Mayo Clinic. Meeting abstract: individualizing Medicine Meeting 2015, Mayo Clinic

Chapter 9

Analysis of Circulating Tumor DNA

Sridurga Mithraprabhu and Andrew Spencer

Abstract

Circulating tumor DNA (ctDNA) analysis is currently gaining momentum as an innovative methodology for characterizing the tumor genome and monitoring therapeutic efficacy in the multifocal, genetically and spatially heterogeneous plasma cell malignancy, multiple myeloma (MM). Circulating cell-free DNA (cfDNA), which consists of a combination of DNA derived from both tumor and normal cells, is present in extracellular bodily fluids. The presence of ctDNA within this admixture has been demonstrated recently in MM. In this chapter, we describe the routinely utilized methodology for the extraction and longitudinal analysis of specific mutations present in ctDNA derived from peripheral blood plasma of MM patients.

Key words Circulating tumor DNA, Circulating cell-free nucleic acids, Cell-free DNA, Multiple myeloma, Peripheral blood plasma, Droplet digital PCR, Liquid biopsy

1 Introduction

The presence of circulating tumor DNA (ctDNA) in extracellular bodily fluids such as plasma, serum, urine, and cerebrospinal fluid enables its evaluation both quantitatively and qualitatively for characterization of the tumor genome and as a biomarker of therapeutic response. The presence of cell free DNA (cfDNA) in body fluids was first described by Mandel and Metais in 1948 [1]. The existence of tumor-derived cfDNA was subsequently observed in cancer patients through the identification of mutated RAS fragments and microsatellite alterations, and critically these alterations were not detected in paired tissue biopsies, emphasizing the concept that isolated tissue biopsies may not represent the optimal material for defining the tumor genome [2, 3]. The more recent development and utilization of next-generation sequencing (NGS) technologies, including whole genome sequencing (WGS), whole exome sequencing (WES), and/or targeted amplicon sequencing (Tam-Seq) of cfDNA, has markedly enhanced the capacity to identify tumor-derived aberrations [4–10]. The advent of these methodologies has resulted in plasma-based analysis for the

Christoph Heuck and Niels Weinhold (eds.), *Multiple Myeloma: Methods and Protocols*, Methods in Molecular Biology, vol. 1792, https://doi.org/10.1007/978-1-4939-7865-6_9,

characterization of potentially targetable oncogenes and the identification of resistance-associated mutations that are acquired during disease progression, thus informing therapeutic changes [5, 11, 12]. Furthermore, the development of various digital PCR applications has enabled the accurate quantification of specific mutations thus allowing longitudinal mutational analysis of sequential plasma or serum samples in patients for monitoring response to therapy [13–18].

The levels of cfDNA in multiple myeloma (MM) patients are significantly higher than in both normal volunteers and non-MM cancers [17, 19]. Moreover, in MM, ctDNA can be detected in plasma and serum with accumulating evidence suggesting that this source material might provide information that cannot be obtained from spatially and temporally restricted bone marrow (BM) aspirates [17, 19–21]. While publications of ctDNA analyses have utilized both plasma and serum, it appears that plasma may provide a superior source for ctDNA analysis, as serum can contain contaminating leukocyte cellular DNA due to clotting factors present in serum collection tubes [22–25]. To enable the further development of ctDNA analysis for clinical benefit including the capacity to compare data derived from multicenter MM studies, it is imperative to establish methodological benchmarks. The isolation, extraction, quantification, and analysis of ctDNA involve multistep methodologies and the use of multiple instruments all of which requires standardization. Several NGS methodologies are available for mutational screening of plasma and the choice of technology needs to be validated within each specific laboratory setting with the procedures for this having been extensively discussed elsewhere [5, 8, 26]. In this chapter we describe the methodologies utilized in our laboratory for longitudinal droplet digital PCR (ddPCR) based analysis of mutations in the peripheral blood plasma ctDNA of MM patients undergoing therapy.

The small quantities of ctDNA in the blood necessitates that contamination from cellular DNA is minimized, and therefore, the type of collection tubes used, the blood storage and transportation conditions, the time between collection to processing and subsequent storage of plasma all needs to be optimized. Unless processing blood samples for plasma within 3 h of blood collection, the usage of EDTA tubes is not recommended, and in our laboratory, Cell-free DNA BCT® tubes (Streck, Omaha, NE) are routinely used. These tubes prevent the lysis of cells through the use of formaldehyde-free reagent thus eliminating/minimising cellular DNA contamination, while protecting against the degradation of cfDNA. Importantly, blood in these tubes can be stored at room temperature until processing [27, 28] that in our laboratory is undertaken within 72 h of blood collection. This thus allows the transportation of samples from potentially geographically distant locations at ambient temperature. Sample processing is then followed by extraction of plasma-derived cfDNA, with the availability of commercial kits having simplified this extraction process while also enabling more high-throughput processing when compared to conventional methods [29]. While a number of commercial kits are available for extraction of cfDNA the QIAGEN circulating nucleic acid kit (QIAamp CNA kit) outperforms most and is routinely utilized with consistent success in our laboratory [29–31]. Following this, the accurate quantitation of extracted cfDNA is critical for determining whether samples have sufficient DNA for subsequent downstream analysis. As such, due to the limited amounts of cfDNA derived and therefore target ctDNA available, it is imperative to utilize methodologies that can reproducibly and with a high-level of accuracy quantify cfDNA. For this purpose, we utilize two methodologies: (1) a QUBIT Fluorometer (Thermo Fisher Scientific, MA, USA) for the quantitation of cfDNA, and then (2) ddPCR (Bio-Rad laboratories, CA, USA) for the measurement of genome equivalents of the reference gene RPP30, which is located on a nonamplifiable region of chromosome 10 [13]. Then, based on the amounts of cfDNA defined by these methods, longitudinal analysis of specific mutations, previously identified with the NGS method of choice, can be performed using ddPCR on sequential plasma samples. As a practical example, ddPCR for three mutations (KRAS G12R, TP53 R372C and NRAS Q61K) in five sequential plasma specimens from the peripheral blood of a relapsed MM patient will be described.

2 Materials

2.1 Blood Collection, Processing and Storage

1. Cell-free DNA BCT® tubes (Streck).
2. Patient peripheral blood.
3. 1.5 mL nuclease-free microcentrifuge tubes.
4. Centrifuge to accommodate 10 mL peripheral blood and 1.5 mL microcentrifuge tubes.
5. Micropipettes and 1 mL nuclease-free sterile filter tips.

2.2 Extraction of cfDNA

1. QIAamp CNA kit (QIAGEN).
2. Proteinase K solution, stored at 4 °C, equilibrated to room temperature.
3. Buffers, solutions and carrier RNA in buffer AL to be prepared and stored as per manufacturers' recommendations.
4. QIAvac 24 plus vacuum manifold, BD Connecta Luer-Lok (Becton Dickinson, NJ, USA) and vacuum pump.
5. Nuclease-free water.
6. 50 mL falcon tubes.

7. 1× phosphate buffered saline (PBS).
8. Shaking water bath at 60 °C.
9. Heat block at 56 °C.
10. Centrifuge.
11. Vortexer.
12. Pipette aspirator and pipettes (5 and 10 mL).
13. Ethanol (96–100%).
14. Micropipette and nuclease-free sterile tips.

2.3 Quantification and Analysis

2.3.1 QUBIT

1. QUBIT 3.0 Fluorometer (Thermo Fisher Scientific).
2. QUBIT dsDNA HS Assay kit (Thermo Fisher Scientific).
3. QUBIT assay tubes (Thermo Fisher Scientific).
4. Tube racks to fit 0.5 mL QUBIT assay tubes.
5. Micropipettes and nuclease-free sterile filter tips.
6. 1.5 mL, 15 mL or 50 mL plastic tube for making up working solution of QUBIT assay HS reagent and buffer.
7. Vortexer.
8. Thawed cfDNA samples.

2.3.2 Droplet Digital PCR (ddPCR)

1. QX200™ Droplet Digital PCR system (Bio-Rad) including automated droplet generator, QX200™ Droplet Reader, C1000 Touch ™ Thermal cycler with 96-deep well reaction module and PX1™ plate sealer.
2. Auto DG consumables including DG32™ automated droplet generator cartridges, auto DG oil for probes, pipet tips, pipet tip waste bin, ddPCR™ 96-well plates. The cooling block accessory as part of the auto DG system should be left at −20 °C at least 1 h prior to droplet generation.
3. ddPCR™ supermix for probes (2×), no dUTP.
4. PCR plate pierceable heat foil.
5. ddPCR™ Droplet Reader Oil.
6. RPP30 Primers and probe (HEX or FAM),

   Forward sequence: AGATTTGGACCTGCGAGCG,

   Reverse sequence: GAGCGGCTGTCTCCACAAGT,

   Probe sequence: TTCTGACCTGAAGGCTCTGCGCG.
7. HaeIII restriction enzyme (RE) 10,000 U/mL (Promega, WI, USA).
8. Micropipettes and nuclease-free sterile filter tips.
9. Nuclease-free PCR grade water.
10. PCR plate centrifuge.

11. Vortexer.
12. cfDNA samples.
13. Positive control DNA.

2.3.3 Longitudinal Mutational Analysis

1. All ddPCR components and experimental setup components from droplet digital PCR section.
2. Extracted and thawed cfDNA samples from five time points.
3. Positive and negative control DNA for KRAS G12R, NRAS Q16K and TP53 R273C.
4. ddPCR™ Primer PCR assays for KRAS G12R, NRAS Q61K and TP53 R273C (Bio-Rad).
5. MseI for KRAS G12R and NRAS Q61K and HaeIII for TP53 R273C (Promega).

3 Methods

3.1 Collection and Isolation of Plasma

1. Collect 8–10 mL of peripheral blood into tubes containing preservative to prevent cellular lysis (*see* **Note 1**).
2. Invert tubes gently 8–10 times to ensure sufficient mixing of bloods with preservative reagent (*see* **Note 2**).
3. Keep at room temperature. All tubes should be kept cool away from sunlight and heat. Tubes can then be transported to processing location (*see* **Note 3**).
4. Centrifuge blood tubes at 820 × *g*, 10 min, ambient temperature.
5. Two layers are distinguished: the upper clear layer is the plasma; a second layer containing a mixed population of white blood cells and erythrocytes.
6. Using a 1 mL pipette and nuclease-free sterile filter tips, carefully aspirate plasma layer from tubes into a sterile 1.5 mL nucleases-free microcentrifuge tube taking care to not disturb the cell layer. Centrifuge at 16,000 × *g*, 10 min at ambient temperature (*see* **Note 4**). Centrifuged samples will contain plasma and pelleted cells.
7. Aspirate supernatant in a new sterile 1.5 mL nuclease-free microcentrifuge tube without dispersing the cell pellet. Store plasma in 1 mL aliquots at −80 °C until further analysis.

3.2 Extraction of cfDNA

In this section, extraction of cfDNA using the QIAamp circulating nucleic acid kit with specific modifications in the manufacturer described protocol "*Purification of Circulating Nucleic Acids from 1 mL, 2 mL, or 3 mL Serum or Plasma*" protocol is described.

1. Thaw plasma samples, equilibrate to room temperature and centrifuge at 16,000 × *g* for 10 min before use (*see* **Note 5**).
2. Heat the water bath and heat block to 60 °C and 56 °C, respectively.
3. Add Proteinase K (300 μL) to a 50 mL centrifuge tube assigned for each sample. Approximately 3 mL of thawed plasma sample can be added to the tube. If less than 3 mL of PL is available, the remainder can be made up with PBS. If less than 3 mL, note the amount of plasma added. This volume will be required for the quantitation of the cfDNA in the sample (Digital PCR for RPP30). Add Buffer ACL containing carrier RNA (2.4 mL) to the tubes, close the cap and pulse-vortex for 30 s. Incubate the tubes in a shaking 60 °C water bath for 30 min (*see* **Note 6**).
4. Add Buffer ACB (5.4 mL) to the tubes, pulse-vortex for 30 s and incubate tubes on ice for 5 min.
5. Assemble the QIAamp mini column into the VacConnector on the QIAvac 24 Plus. Insert the tube extender into the mini-column and carefully transfer the contents of the tube to the tube extender and switch on the vacuum. Carefully discard the tube extender while retaining the column once all plasma–buffer mixture is drawn through (*see* **Note 7**). Switch off the vacuum.
6. Apply buffer ACW1 (600 μL) to the mini-column and switch on vacuum to drain the buffer through. Follow this with the addition of 750 μL of Buffer ACW2 and switch on vacuum until the buffer is drained.
7. Add Ethanol (100%, 750 μL) to the mini-column and switch on vacuum. Once the ethanol has drawn through, switch off vacuum. The mini-column lids should be closed before removing from the vacuum. Place in clean 2 mL collection tubes.
8. Centrifuge mini-columns at 20,000 × *g* for 3 min at room temperature and then place in clean 2 mL collection tubes.
9. Open the lids of the mini-columns and incubate in the heat block at 56 °C for 10 min to dry out the membrane.
10. Place the mini-columns in 1.5 mL microcentrifuge nuclease-free sterile tubes. Apply 100 μL of Buffer AVE to the center of the membranes, close lids, and incubate at room temperature for 3 min (*see* **Note 8**).
11. Centrifuge at 20,000 × *g* for 1 min to elute the cfDNA. The samples should be stored at −80 °C until required.

3.3 Quantitation

3.3.1 QUBIT Fluorometer

1. The concentration of cfDNA in the elution is quantitated using the Qubit 3.0 Fluorometer and the Qubit dsDNA HS (double-stranded DNA high sensitivity) Assay kit.

2. Make enough working solution of Qubit dsDNA HS dye in buffer in a plastic tube (1:200 ratio) to accommodate both samples and two standards. A total of 200 μL DNA–working solution is required for each sample.
3. To generate the two standards, add 10 μL of each QUBIT standard (Standard 1 and 2, components C and D, 1 and 10 ng/μL, respectively) to 190 μL of working solution in 0.5 mL tubes QUBIT assay tubes. Mix standards by vortexing for 2–3 s and reserve. Prepare standards fresh for every use.
4. Use 5 μL of cfDNA elution to 195 μL of working solution (*see* **Note 9**). Vortex tubes for 2–3 s and incubate at room temperature for 2 min.
5. On the QUBIT Fluorometer 3.0 home screen, choose dsDNA and High sensitivity assays.
6. Press "Read standards." Run a new calibration for standards every time using the generated standards. Following the prompts, insert "standard 1" (0 ng/μL) and press read. Insert "standard 2" (10 ng/μL) and press read.
7. Once the standards have been read, the system will display the calibration readings and will allow for reading of the samples.
8. Before reading the actual samples, read standard 2 as your first sample (*see* **Note 10**). Choose the sample volume as 10 μL for this measurement.
9. Choose the sample volume as 5 μL for reading the samples. Press "read sample" and the concentration of the sample will be displayed. Proceed to read the rest of the samples (*see* **Notes 9** and **11**). Record the concentration of the samples.

3.3.2 Droplet Digital PCR

1. Thaw all components to be used for ddPCR. Mix the reagents thoroughly using a vortex and briefly centrifuge to collect content of the tubes to the bottom.
2. Based on the number of reactions required, a master mix should be prepared without the addition of the sample template. For quantitation assays, duplicates of each sample are recommended. Include a positive control and a negative nuclease-free dH20 control in duplicates for RPP30 primer assay.
3. The PCR mastermix comprises a mixture of the 2× ddPCR supermix for probes, RPP30 primers and probes, restriction enzyme HaeIII, and nuclease-free water. A 22 μL final reaction volume is to be loaded in each well of the PCR plate for the auto DG. However, to account for pipetting errors, a 25 μL volume should be made (Table 1, *see* **Note 12**). The use of HaeIII is recommended for this ddPCR assay as it provides better separation between the positive and the negative droplets (Fig. 1).

Table 1
Reagent setup for quantitative assessment of RPP30 in cfDNA samples

Reagent	Volume (for 25 μL)
2× ddPCR supermix for probes, no dUTP	12.5 μL
20× primers/probe (HEX or FAM)	1.25 μL
Restriction enzyme, HaeIII (10,000 U/mL)—diluted to 2 U (*see* **Note 13**)	0.2 μL
Nuclease-free water	11.05
cfDNA sample	2 μL

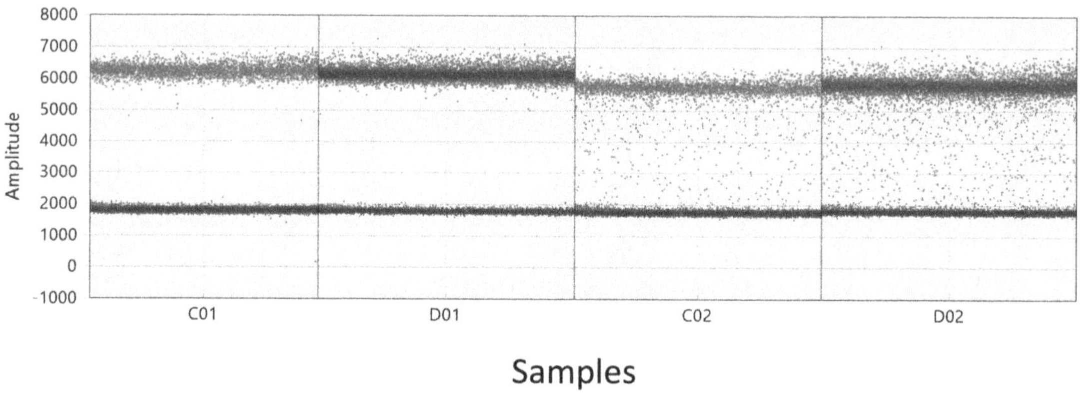

Fig. 1 RPP30 assay was performed in samples with and without restriction enzyme HaeIII. The plot shows the droplets (positive and negative event numbers) vs. fluorescence amplitude in samples with HaeIII (C01 and D01) and without HaeIII (C02 and D02). The addition of HaeIII provides better separation of the positive droplets (green) from the negative droplets (grey)

4. Once master mix components are added, briefly vortex and centrifuge to collect all reagents to the bottom of the tube.
5. Dispense 23 μL of this master mix in PCR plates calculating for duplicates of samples, positive and negative controls (*see* **Note 14**).
6. Add 2 μL of each sample to the aliquoted mastermix. Mix thoroughly (8–10 times) and briefly centrifuge (*see* **Note 15**). Allow the samples to equilibrate at ambient temperature for 5 min.
7. Set the PX1 plate sealer to seal plates at 180 °C for 5 s. Allow the plate sealer to reach the desired temperature. Touch the arrow to open the PX1 tray door, place the 96-well block, and position the plate onto the support block. Place one sheet of the pierceable heat seal with the red line face-up, ensuring that it covers the plate properly and press the "Seal" button.

The tray will close and open automatically once the plates are sealed (*see* **Note 16**). Proceed to droplet generation.

8. Power on the auto DG to allow self-check of the instrument. The touch screen menu will have a layout of the instrument deck highlighted in grey indicating that consumables need to be loaded. Touch the "Configure Sample Plate" button on the screen, select the number of columns in which samples are located by touching the columns. Enter plate names or notes, if required and click "OK." Once the number of columns has been selected, the auto DG screen will blink yellow to indicate positions on the instrument deck where the consumables should be loaded.
9. Load the auto DG with consumables working from backward to avoid contamination. Place the DG32 cartridge plates with the green gaskets toward the right. Each DG32 cartridge has four 8-well columns, therefore, load plates according to the number of samples prepared. When the DG32 cartridge plate is loaded correctly, the lights will turn green from yellow, both on the touch screen and in the plate holders.
10. Load the auto DG pipette tips after opening the box lids in the middle area of the instrument deck. Make sure there are enough tips for all samples (*see* **Note 17**). The corresponding lights will turn green. Load a new waste bin.
11. Load the sealed PCR plate into the front left plate holder, labeled as "Sample Plate" on the touch screen. The plate will fit only in the right orientation and the lights on the sample plate holder and screen will turn green when properly installed.
12. Assemble the cooled block and place into the front right plate holder, which is indicated as the "Droplet plate" on the screen. If properly cooled, the block will turn to purple from pink. A cooled block prevents the droplets from evaporating. Once the block is placed, the light will turn green. Place a fresh PCR plate on the block in the proper orientation (*see* **Note 18**).
13. Remove the cap of the droplet generation oil bottle, twist on the bottle until it stops into the tower of the oil delivery system at the front left corner of the instrument. If loaded right, the label on the bottle will face out.
14. Select the oil type as "Probe". Once the icon on the screen turns blue, the current level of the oil will be displayed. The tower light will turn green.
15. When all consumables are loaded, the touch screen "Start" icon will turn blue. Pressing the "Start" button will bring up a summary screen of the setup, confirm if entered details are accurate and touch the "Start Run" button. Once the run has started, the auto DG doors will close automatically and should

Table 2
Cycling conditions for ddPCR assay on C1000 Touch™ Thermocycler

Step	Temperature in °C	Time	Ramp rate	Number of cycles
Enzyme activation	95	10 min	2 °C/s	1
Denaturation	94	30 s		40
Annealing/extension (*see* **Note 19**)	55	1 min		
Enzyme deactivation	98	10 min		1
Hold	4	Infinite	1 °C/s	1

remain closed until all droplets are generated. The touch screen will display the time remaining until the droplets are ready. When "Droplets ready" message is displayed, the doors will unlock and the plate can be removed.

16. Seal the PCR plate with the PX1 plate sealer, as before.
17. Proceed to PCR reaction immediately.
18. Switch on the C1000 Touch™ Thermal cycler and program the cycling conditions (Table 2).
19. Place the PCR plate in the thermal cycler for PCR amplification.
20. Set the reaction volume to 40 μL and use the heated lid option when starting the PCR run.
21. Following PCR, the plates can be stored at 4 °C for up to 1 week. We recommend reading the droplets immediately.
22. Read the droplets with the QX200 Droplet reader.
23. For setting the plate layout, open the QuantaSoft software, click the "Setup" and choose the absolute quantification and the ddPCR supermix for probes (no dUTP) setting (QuantaSoft software instruction manual, 10031906).
24. Double click the well to enter all information including sample and target name (RPP30), channel (Ch2 for HEX or Ch1 for FAM) and whether it is unknown concentration, positive or negative control. Select "Apply" to load the wells.
25. Once all information is entered, click "Run" to start the analysis. Select the dye set and run options. Each sample takes approximately 2 min to read.
26. When the run is completed, click the "Analyze." There are five tabs within the analysis window, including 1D amplitude, 2D amplitude, concentration, copy number, ratio and droplets. Check the number of droplets in each well. A minimum of 10,000 droplets is required for the well to be included in the sample analysis.

27. Next, check the threshold setting using the 1D amplitude plot. The threshold should be set manually taking into consideration the fluorescence amplitude in the positive and negative samples (Fig. 1). After setting the threshold for all sample wells, we recommend manually checking each sample to determine if the settings are appropriate.
28. The "Concentration" tab provides the concentration of the RPP30 DNA molecule in the sample as copies/μL. This value indicates the number of copies in 20 μL of the reaction.
29. The amount of copies per volume of plasma can be calculated from this value. For example, if there were 10 copies/μL and a total of 25 μL of the PCR mix was made, then a total of 10 × 25 = 250 copies of RPP30 is present in the PCR mix. Since, 2 μL of the sample was added into the reaction mix, 250/2 = 125 copies/μL of RPP30 was present in the starting material. Therefore, if 3 mL of plasma sample was used for extraction and cfDNA was eluted in 100 μL volume, 100 × 125 = 12,500 copies are present in total. Finally, 12,500/3 = 4166.7 copies of RPP30 is present in 1 mL peripheral blood plasma in this patient. This standardized value can be used to compare the amounts of cfDNA between samples (*see* **Note 20**).

3.4 Longitudinal Mutational Analysis

1. Thaw all components of ddPCR reaction set up, as before. Set up the reaction according to Table 3. All samples should be run in quadruples to optimize the sensitivity of the experiment for the detection of rare mutations.
2. The amounts of cfDNA in each sample should be diluted to approximately the same amount for longitudinal assessment of ctDNA copies (*see* **Note 21**).

Table 3
Reagent set up for longitudinal assessment of mutations using HEX for reference and FAM for the target mutation with ddPCR

Reagent	Volume (for 25 μL)
2× ddPCR supermix for probes, no dUTP	12.5 μL
20× primers/probe (FAM), target assay	1.25 μL
20× primers/probe (HEX), reference assay	1.25 μL
Restriction enzyme, diluted to 2 U (*see* **Note 13**)	0.2 μL
Nuclease-free water	4.8 μL
cfDNA sample	5 μL

3. Once master mix components are added, proceed to PCR plate set up, droplet generation and PCR amplification, as before.
4. Read the droplets with the QX200 Droplet reader.
5. For setting the plate layout, open the QuantaSoft software, click the "Setup" and choose the "Rare event detection" and the ddPCR supermix for probes (no dUTP) setting.
6. Double click the well to enter all information including sample and target name, reference name and whether it is unknown concentration, positive, negative or no-template control. Select "Apply" to load the wells. Perform run as before.
7. When the run is completed, check the number of droplets in each well. A minimum of 10,000 droplets is required for the well to be included in the sample analysis.
8. Next, check the threshold setting using the 1D and 2D amplitude plot. The threshold should be set manually taking into consideration the fluorescence amplitude in the positive samples making sure there are no droplets in the negative control or no-template control. A clear separation of negative droplets, FAM+ (target only), HEX+ (reference only) and double positive cells should be observed (*see* **Note 22**). A representative example of threshold settings using KRAS G12R positive control is shown in Fig. 2. Select all samples with the specific mutation assay and set thresholds accordingly.
9. For rare event detection, samples that have more than three positive droplets across the four wells are taken as positive, if the negative control sample has no positive droplets (*see* **Note 22**).
10. The "Concentration" tab provides the concentration of the copies/μL. This, as before, can be utilized to calculate the copies in certain amount of starting material.
11. The "Ratio" tab provides the fractional abundance of the sample, which is a ratio of the *Mutation/(Wildtype + Mutation)* to determine if the measured fractional abundance of mutants is the expected amount. Record the fractional abundance of mutant copies relative to wild type copies using the "merged wells" setting, which takes into account droplets across the four replicates of each sample. A representative example of TP53 R273 fractional abundance for the sequential plasma samples from the QuantaSoft software is shown (Fig. 3).
12. Fractional abundance values can be sequentially plotted and correlated to the treatment the patient was receiving at any particular time. The fractional abundance of KRAS G12R, TP53 R273C, and NRAS Q61K in sequential plasma specimens collected over a period of 45 months along with the

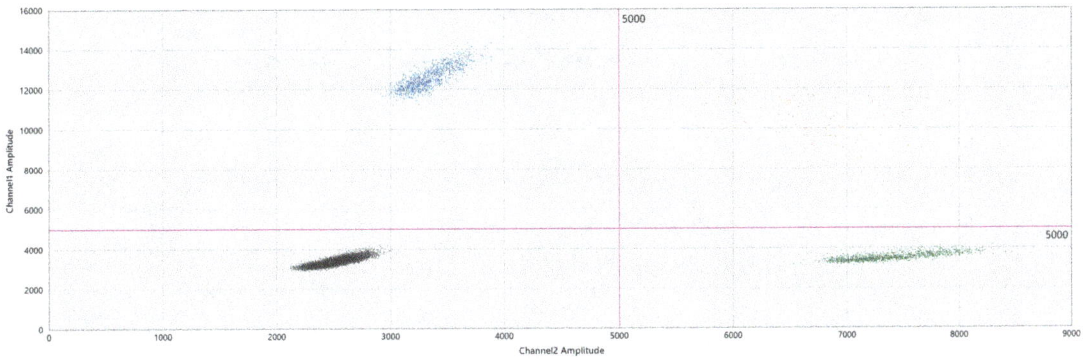

Fig. 2 A 2D-amplitude plot showing droplets that are positive for FAM (channel 1, blue) or HEX (channel 2, green), double positive (orange) or negative (grey). The threshold should be set in a manner that allows for clear demarcation of the four different populations as represented by the pink lines

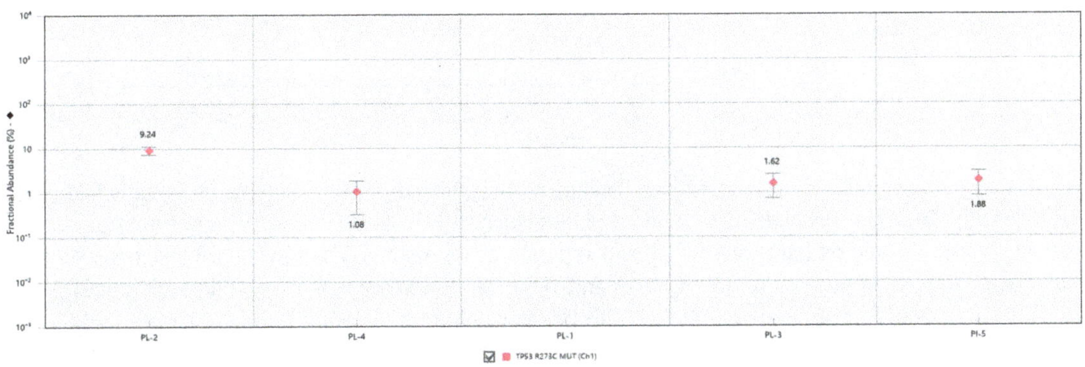

Fig. 3 Fractional abundance plot of TP53 R273C in sequential plasma specimens

serum-free light chain concentration (biomarker of tumor burden in MM patients) in a relapsed MM patient undergoing therapy are shown in Fig. 4.

4 Notes

1. It is not always possible to collect 8–10 mL per tube as this depends on the patient circumstances. Additionally, under certain circumstances more than 10 mL of blood might be required from a patient to ensure enough material is available for all types of downstream analysis. Less than 8 mL per tube will not be economical, however, it is adequate for analysis.
2. Proper mixing of blood with preservative ensures stabilization and should be performed. Collection tubes with preservative will have a defined shelf-life and it is important to use tubes within this shelf-life.

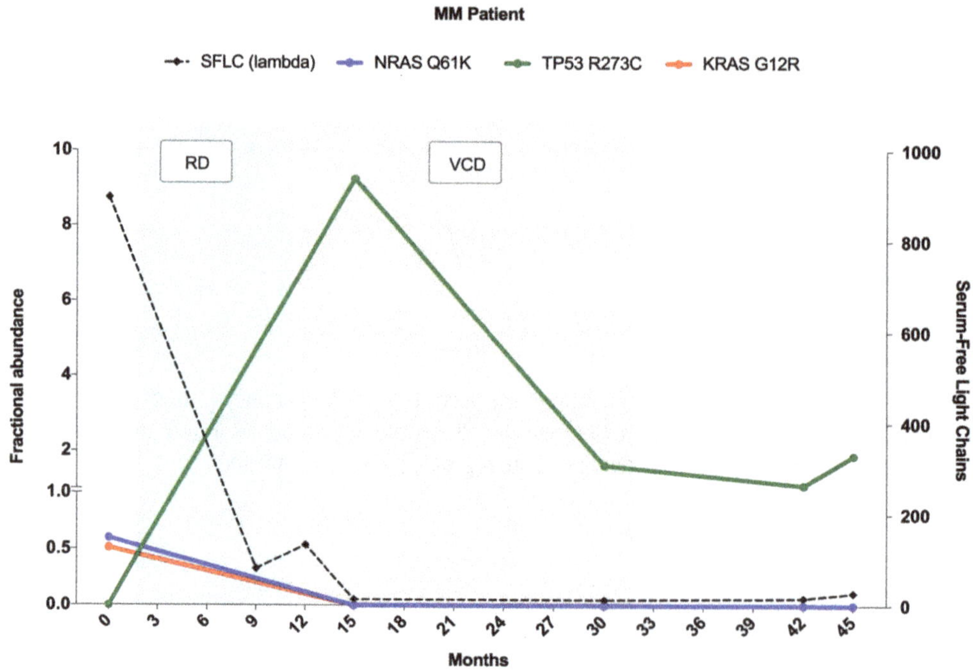

Fig. 4 A MM patient with advanced relapsed disease had sequential plasma samples collected while being treated with Revlimid (lenalidomide) and dexamethasone (RD) followed by Velcade (bortezomib)—Cyclophosphamide—Dexamethasone (VCD) over a period of 45 months. The fractional abundance of three mutations, KRAS G12R (red), NRAS Q61K (blue) and TP53 R273C (green) was assessed utilizing ddCPR. The fractional abundance values were correlated with the concentration of serum-free light chains (SFLC). MM harboring the KRAS G12R and NRAS Q61K mutations was responsive to RD; however, the SFLC increased in unison with the emergence of a different RD-resistant TP53 R273C positive MM clone necessitating a change of therapy to VCD. Following this, both the SFLC concentration and TP53 R273C levels decreased. Importantly, while SFLC levels normalized, the TP53 R273C mutant ctDNA remained readily detectable in the plasma

3. It is advisable to use plastic tubes instead of glass to prevent breakage during transport. Most commercial companies that offer cfDNA compatible collection tubes currently have plastic tubes.
4. It is critical to do two spins (one lower and one higher) to ensure removal of cell pellet, platelets and debris and for efficient recovery of cell-free plasma.
5. This step ensures removal of remnant debris in the plasma. This is critical to ensure that there is no blockage in the spin column when the vacuum manifold is utilized.
6. A shaking water bath ensures that plasma:buffer mixture is consistently mixed to ensure optimal digestion of contaminating proteins and nucleases.
7. The vacuum should be on until all the buffer had drawn through. For 3 mL of input plasma, the mixture should pass through the vacuum in approximately 10 min. However, if there are samples that are delayed, then ensure that samples

that are done are not sitting in the vacuum for more than 5 min. If so, proceed with the isolation using buffer ACW1 and subsequent steps using centrifuge. The centrifuge spin should be at >8000 × *g*, 5 min, ambient temperature. For delayed samples, if mixture does not pass through completely after 30 min since commencing the vacuum, remove samples and manually centrifuge in 750 μL aliquots using the mini-column at >8000 × *g*, 5 min, ambient temperature. Continue until all of the plasma:buffer mixture is finished. Subsequent steps to be performed accordingly. The recently launched QIAGEN ccfDNA kit appears to have solved the issue of vacuum blockage, thus eliminating the need to stagger isolation arising out of delay in plasma:buffer mixture flow through.

8. Elution volume should be standardized across all sample extractions. A 100 μL elution volume appears to be sufficient for downstream analysis. If a higher concentration of cfDNA is required, a 50 μL elution volume can also be utilized.
9. Usually, a 5 μL amount of cfDNA is enough for a majority of the samples. If the amount is undetectable on QUBIT, this volume can be increased up to 20 μL. This requires 180 μL of the QUBIT HS reagent and buffer working solution to make a final volume of 200 μL.
10. Using a commercially available standard at a certain ng/μL (in this case 10 ng/μL) will determine if the standard, the instrument or the sample preparation is at fault. The concentration of this should be close to the expected value.
11. If the sample concentration is displayed as "out of range" (too high), prepare another dilution of the sample with the working solution using a volume that is less than 5 μL. Usually, a 2 μL sample input is appropriate in these instances.
12. Auto DG requires 22 μL of mastermix–DNA template. We recommend making up a little more, between 23 and 25 μL to ensure enough sample is available for loading into the automated droplet generator. A 23 μL volume is both optimal and economical, provided pipettes are calibrated and pipetting is accurate.
13. An aliquot of the restriction enzyme can be added without diluting depending on the number of samples. For example, for a 2 U addition per reaction from a 10,000 U/mL stock, a 0.2 μL is required for one reaction. If making a mastermix for 10 samples, this amount to 2 μL of the restriction enzyme, which can be added directly.
14. The ddPCR set up works well in multiples of eight. If less than that, make up the rest of the PCR plate with blank control tubes (QX200 Buffer control kit for probes). However, we recommend that samples are set up in such a way that all wells are utilized for sample analysis.

15. A homogenous sample is mandatory for optimal ddPCR analysis.
16. Check if the impression of the well outline is seen once the plate is sealed. Improper sealing will result in the droplets evaporating during the PCR reaction.
17. Each sample will use two tips, one for aspirating the sample and one for dispensing the generated droplets.
18. Do not forget to load a clean PCR plate into the block. As the light turns green as soon as the cooled block is placed, irrespective of whether a PCR plate is fitted or not, the possibility of starting the run without a PCR plate for the droplets is high. To avoid this, always load the clean PCR plate on the cooled block before assembling on the instrument deck.
19. For the RPP30 primer/probe set up, a temperature gradient PCR to check the optimal annealing temperature was performed. It is recommended that each laboratory perform the temperature gradient PCR to identify the optimal temperature.
20. The values of RPP30 should be correlated to the QUBIT concentrations to determine uniformity between the two methodologies.
21. Copy numbers of RPP30 in the starting material was calculated according to instructions in the quantitation section and the samples were equilibrated using nuclease-free water to contain approximately the same number of copies. Equal amounts of the diluted samples were used for ddPCR mutational analysis. The amounts of DNA in the positive and negative control samples should be preferably equal or more than the test samples.
22. If positive droplets are seen in the negative control samples, these positive droplets should be taken into consideration. For detailed guidelines on how to calculate the false positive rate of each sample, refer to the "Bio-Rad ddPCR Rare Mutation Detection Best Practices Guidelines".

References

1. Mandel P, Metais P (1948) Les acides nucléiques du plasma sanguin chez l'homme. C R Seances Soc Biol Fil 142(3–4):241–243
2. Chen XQ et al (1996) Microsatellite alterations in plasma DNA of small cell lung cancer patients. Nat Med 2(9):1033–1035
3. Vasioukhin V et al (1994) Point mutations of the N-ras gene in the blood plasma DNA of patients with myelodysplastic syndrome or acute myelogenous leukaemia. Br J Haematol 86(4):774–779
4. Chan KC et al (2013) Cancer genome scanning in plasma: detection of tumor-associated copy number aberrations, single-nucleotide variants, and tumoral heterogeneity by massively parallel sequencing. Clin Chem 59(1):211–224
5. Forshew T et al (2012) Noninvasive identification and monitoring of cancer mutations by targeted deep sequencing of plasma DNA. Sci Transl Med 4(136):136–168
6. Heitzer E et al (2013) Tumor-associated copy number changes in the circulation of patients

with prostate cancer identified through whole-genome sequencing. Genome Med 5(4):30

7. Leary RJ et al (2012) Detection of chromosomal alterations in the circulation of cancer patients with whole-genome sequencing. Sci Transl Med 4(162):162–154
8. Murtaza M et al (2013) Non-invasive analysis of acquired resistance to cancer therapy by sequencing of plasma DNA. Nature 497(7447):108–112
9. Plagnol V et al. (2015) Assessment of clinical applications of circulating tumor DNA using an enhanced TAm-Seq platform. J Clin Oncol. 33(15)
10. Kidess E et al (2015) Mutation profiling of tumor DNA from plasma and tumor tissue of colorectal cancer patients with a novel, high-sensitivity multiplexed mutation detection platform. Oncotarget 6(4):2549–2561
11. Demetri GD et al (2013) Mutational analysis of plasma DNA from patients (pts) in the phase III GRID study of regorafenib (REC) versus placebo (PL) in tyrosine kinase inhibitor (TKI)-refractory GIST: correlating genotype with clinical outcomes. J Clin Oncol 31(15):10503
12. Demetri GD, et al. (2013) Detection of oncogenic kinase mutations in circulating plasma DNA and correlation with clinical benefit in the phase III GRID study of regorafenib vs placebo in TKI-refractory metastatic GIST. Cancer Res. 73(8)
13. Dawson SJ et al (2013) Analysis of circulating tumor DNA to monitor metastatic breast cancer. N Engl J Med 368(13):1199–1209
14. Tsao SC et al (2015) Monitoring response to therapy in melanoma by quantifying circulating tumor DNA with droplet digital PCR for BRAF and NRAS mutations. Sci Rep 5:11198
15. Olsson E et al (2015) Serial monitoring of circulating tumor DNA in patients with primary breast cancer for detection of occult metastatic disease. EMBO Mol Med 7(8):1034–1047
16. Oxnard GR et al (2014) Noninvasive detection of response and resistance in EGFR-mutant lung cancer using quantitative next-generation genotyping of cell-free plasma DNA. Clin Cancer Res 20(6):1698–1705
17. Mithraprabhu S et al (2017) Circulating tumor DNA analysis demonstrates spatial mutational heterogeneity that coincides with disease relapse in myeloma. Leukemia 31(8):1695–1705
18. Sanmamed MF et al (2015) Quantitative cell-free circulating BRAFV600E mutation analysis by use of droplet digital PCR in the follow-up of patients with melanoma being treated with BRAF inhibitors. Clin Chem 61(1):297–304
19. Kis O et al (2017) Circulating tumor DNA sequence analysis as an alternative to multiple myeloma bone marrow aspirates. Nat Commun 8:15086
20. Rustad EH et al (2017) Monitoring multiple myeloma by quantification of recurrent mutations in serum. Haematologica 102(7):1266–1272
21. Oberle A et al (2017) Monitoring multiple myeloma by next-generation sequencing of V(D)J rearrangements from circulating myeloma cells and cell-free myeloma DNA. Haematologica 102(6):1105–1111
22. Jen J, Wu L, Sidransky D (2000) An overview on the isolation and analysis of circulating tumor DNA in plasma and serum. Ann N Y Acad Sci 906:8–12
23. Jung M et al (2003) Changes in concentration of DNA in serum and plasma during storage of blood samples. Clin Chem 49(6 Pt 1):1028–1029
24. Lee TH et al (2001) Quantitation of genomic DNA in plasma and serum samples: higher concentrations of genomic DNA found in serum than in plasma. Transfusion 41(2):276–282
25. Umetani N, Hiramatsu S, Hoon DS (2006) Higher amount of free circulating DNA in serum than in plasma is not mainly caused by contaminated extraneous DNA during separation. Ann N Y Acad Sci 1075:299–307
26. Ulz P, Auer M, Heitzer E (2016) Detection of circulating tumor DNA in the blood of cancer patients: an important tool in cancer chemoprevention. Methods Mol Biol 1379:45–68
27. Norton SE et al (2013) A stabilizing reagent prevents cell-free DNA contamination by cellular DNA in plasma during blood sample storage and shipping as determined by digital PCR. Clin Biochem 46(15):1561–1565
28. Norton SE et al (2013) A new blood collection device minimizes cellular DNA release during sample storage and shipping when compared to a standard device. J Clin Lab Anal 27(4):305–311
29. Fong SL et al (2009) Comparison of 7 methods for extracting cell-free DNA from serum samples of colorectal cancer patients. Clin Chem 55(3):587–589
30. Devonshire AS et al (2014) Towards standardisation of cell-free DNA measurement in plasma: controls for extraction efficiency, fragment size bias and quantification. Anal Bioanal Chem 406(26):6499–6512
31. Mauger F et al (2015) Comprehensive evaluation of methods to isolate, quantify, and characterize circulating cell-free DNA from small volumes of plasma. Anal Bioanal Chem 407(22):6873–6878

Chapter 10

Detection of Cross-Sample Contamination in Multiple Myeloma Samples and Sequencing Data

Owen W. Stephens, Tobias Meißner, and Niels Weinhold

Abstract

The increasing applicability and sensitivity of next generation sequencing methods exacerbate one of the main issues in the molecular biology laboratory, namely cross-sample contamination. This type of contamination, which could massively increase the rate of false-positive calls in sequencing experiments, can originate at each step during the processing of multiple myeloma samples, such as CD138-selection of tumor cells, RNA and DNA isolation or the processing of sequencing libraries. Here we describe a Droplet Digital PCR (ddPCR) method and a simple bioinformatic solution for the detection of contamination in patient's samples and derived sequencing data, which are based on the same principle: detection of alternative alleles for single-nucleotide polymorphisms (SNPs) that are homozygous according to the control (germ line) sample.

Key words Multiple myeloma, Cross-sample contamination, SNP-based assay, Droplet digital PCR, Bioinformatics solution

1 Introduction

Advances in genome-wide DNA and RNA profiling methods, especially the introduction of next generation sequencing based approaches, have significantly improved our understanding of the plasma cell disease multiple myeloma (MM) [1–4]. These methods have brought many opportunities that were once unattainable with standard molecular techniques. The recent introduction of single-cell techniques has further extended the spectrum of methods and these methods do not only allow for the analysis of single tumor cells but will also lead to a better understanding of the complex cell-cell interactions within the tumor microenvironment [5, 6].

However, the increasing applicability and sensitivity of these "next-generation" methods exacerbate one of the main issues in the molecular biology laboratory, namely cross-sample

Owen W. Stephens and Tobias Meißner contributed equally to this work.

Christoph Heuck and Niels Weinhold (eds.), *Multiple Myeloma: Methods and Protocols*, Methods in Molecular Biology, vol. 1792, https://doi.org/10.1007/978-1-4939-7865-6_10, © Springer Science+Business Media, LLC, part of Springer Nature 2018

contamination. This type of contamination, which could massively increase the rate of false-positive calls in sequencing experiments, can originate at each step during the processing of MM samples, such as CD138-selection of tumor cells, RNA and DNA isolation or the processing of sequencing libraries. It is well known that the initial preanalytical phase is most error prone when samples become labeled, identified, or aliquoted. But once a sample goes through the preanalytical stage, it is often difficult to track sample mishandling. This holds true especially for "old" samples in bio-banks that might not have been processed with procedures that meet today's standards.

Here we describe a Droplet Digital PCR (ddPCR) method and a simple bioinformatic solution for detection of contamination in patient's samples and sequencing data, respectively, which are based on the same principle: detection of alternative alleles for single-nucleotide polymorphisms (SNPs) that are homozygous according to the control (germ line) sample (Fig. 1). For a SNP-based assay the following criteria have to be fulfilled: (i) SNPs not in linkage disequilibrium, (ii) high variant allele frequency (VAF), and (iii) low variation in the VAF between different ethnic groups [7]. For ddPCR we considered SNPs from two previously described panels [8, 9]. We filtered for SNPs located on the commonly aberrant chromosomes in MM and selected a set of 15 SNPs (Table 1). This simple set was optimized for effort and cost per sample. Since we use the Biomark HD for initial genotyping of patients, we usually genotype the first 12 SNPs in Table 1. If less than four SNPs are homozygous per patient, we also genotype the remaining three SNPs in another run. For the bioinformatic solution we increased the discriminatory power by including a set of 200 SNPs using the software program called "SNP_Tagger" [7]. While the lab-based method can be applied at every phase of sample handling and adds another layer of quality assurance in the molecular biology laboratory at a modest cost, the bioinformatics approach allows for an effective detection of contamination and sample mix-up in existing DNA and RNA sequencing data.

2 Material

2.1 Genotyping of Patients

1. Flex Six IFC (Fluidigm).
2. Biomark HD (Fluidigm).
3. Juno (Fluidigm).
4. 2× Assay Loading Reagent (Fluidigm).
5. ROX Reference Dye (50×).
6. SNP Genotyping Assay Mix (40×).
7. TaqMan Universal PCR Master Mix (Life Technologies).

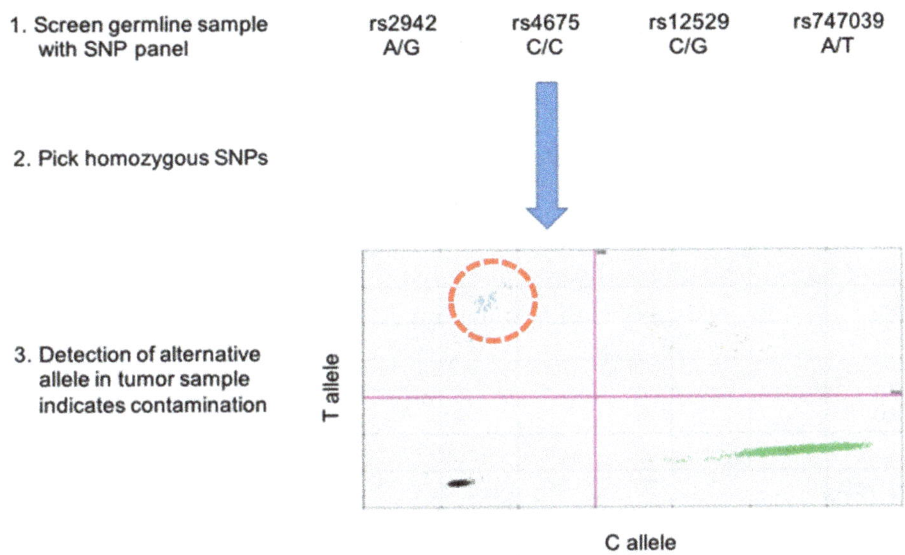

Fig. 1 Approach to assess cross-sample contamination. The droplet Digital PCR (ddPCR) method and the bioinformatic solution for detection of contamination are based on the same principle: detection of alternative alleles for single-nucleotide polymorphisms (SNPs) that are homozygous according to the control (germ line) sample. The figure shows the result of a ddPCR for SNP rs4675 in a tumor sample as an example. The SNP was homozygous C/C in the germ line sample. Detection of the alternative T allele indicated contamination. Heterozygous signals are due to droplets containing more than one copy of the respective DNA locus

8. 20× Fast GT Sample Loading Reagent (Fluidigm).
9. AmpliTaq Gold DNA Polymerase (Life Technologies).
10. Molecular grade water.
11. DNA from control (germ line) sample with a concentration of 10 ng/μL.

2.2 Detection of Contamination by Droplet Digital PCR

1. QX100 Droplet Digital PCR System (Bio-Rad).
2. Droplet Generation Oil for Probes (Bio-Rad).
3. DG8 Cartridges for QX100 Droplet Generator (Bio-Rad).
4. DG8 Gaskets for QX100 Droplet Generator (Bio-Rad).
5. 96-well thermal cycler.
6. 96-well PCR plates, semiskirted.
7. ddPCR Supermix for Probes (Bio-Rad).
8. Pierceable Foil Heat Seal (Fisher).
9. DNA from tumor sample with a concentration of 10 ng/μL.

2.3 Detection of Contamination in Sequencing Data

1. Sequencing data of normal and tumor samples aligned to the human genome reference GRCh37 (*see* **Notes 1** and **2**).
2. R/Bioconductor installation (r-project.org/bioconductor.org).

3. R/Bioconductor packages/dependencies

   Optparse.

   Rsamtools.

   VariantAnnotation.

   GenomicRanges.

   plyr.

4. Contamination detection script (https://github.com/NWeinh/Contamination_Detection).

3 Methods

3.1 Genotyping of Patients

1. Prime the Flex Six IFC according to the manufacturer's instruction (*see* **Note 3**).
2. For each of the first 12 assays in Table 1 prepare a 10× assay mix stock by combining 25 μL 2× Assay Loading Reagent, 2.5 μL ROX™ Reference Dye (50×), 10 μL molecular grade water, and 12.5 μL SNP Genotyping Assay Mix (40×) (*see* **Note 4**).

Table 1
Panel for droplet digital PCR

SNP	Allele/fluorophore	Build 37 location	Assay ID	MAF
rs2942	(*A* = VIC/*G* = FAM)	Chr6:146755140	C_175678541_10	*G* = 0.47
rs4675	(*C* = VIC/*T* = FAM)	Chr22:21141300	C__3269373_30	*T* = 0.48
rs12529	(*C* = VIC/*G* = FAM)	Chr10:5136651	C__8723970_1_	*C* = 0.42
rs747039	(*A* = VIC/*G* = FAM)	Chr17:47406913	C__1121246_10	*G* = 0.39
rs7300444	(*C* = VIC/*T* = FAM)	Chr12:993930	C__1244577_10	*T* = 0.40
rs9962023	(*C* = VIC/*T* = FAM)	Chr18:21413869	C_25593660_20	*T* = 0.38
rs10203363	(*C* = VIC/*T* = FAM)	Chr2:227896976	C_22273357_10	*T* = 0.50
rs12997453	(*A* = VIC/*G* = FAM)	Chr2:182413259	C__1276208_10	*A* = 0.35
rs10883099	(*A* = VIC/*G* = FAM)	Chr10:100219314	C__9589522_10	*G* = 0.47
rs1019029	(*A* = VIC/*G* = FAM)	Chr7:13894276	C__2572254_10	*A* = 0.48
rs1410059	(*C* = VIC/*T* = FAM)	Chr10:97172595	C__7538108_10	*T* = 0.41
rs521861	(*C* = VIC/*G* = FAM)	Chr18:47371014	C__2714437_1_	*G* = 0.49
rs1034178	(*C* = VIC/*T* = FAM)	Chr10:106899421	C__1367957_1_	*C* = 0.47
rs9951171	(*A* = VIC/*G* = FAM)	Chr18:9749879	C__1371205_10	*A* = 0.45
rs3780962	(*A* = VIC/*G* = FAM)	Chr10:17193346	C__2822618_10	*A* = 0.50

3. Prepare the sample premix for one partition (12 assays per sample) by mixing 45 μL 2× TaqMan® Universal PCR Master, 4.5 μL 20× GT Sample Loading Reagent, 0.9 μL AmpliTaq Gold® DNA Polymerase, and 2.1 μL molecular grade water.
4. Mix 3.5 μL of sample premix with 2.5 μL DNA sample.
5. Load the Flex Six IFC with the assay mix and the sample premix and collect the genotyping data using the run scripts "One Step Flex Six" and "Standard: Collect End-Point Data" according to the manufacturer's instruction (*see* **Note 3**). Store unused assay mix at −20 °C for up to 3 weeks.
6. Determine the genotype of SNPs.
7. Genotype the three remaining SNPs in Table 1, if less than four SNPs are homozygous per patient.

3.2 Detection of Contamination by Droplet Digital PCR

1. From the initial genotyping experiment, select four homozygous SNPs per patient (*see* **Note 5**).
2. Per patient sample and SNP, prepare a reaction mix in a tube of an 8-tube PCR strip by mixing:

   9.4 μL nuclease-free water.

   12.5 μL 2× Supermix.

   0.6 μL 40× Taqman assay.

   2.5 μL DNA (10 ng/μL).
3. Load a droplet generator cartridge into the cartridge holder.
4. Gently pipette the reaction mixture up and down using a multichannel pipettor (*see* **Note 6**).
5. Per sample, transfer 20 μL of the reaction mixture to a well of the middle row of the droplet generator cartridge ("Sample" row) (*see* **Note 7**).
6. Fill unused wells with 20 μL of 1× ddPCR buffer control.
7. Remove any bubbles in the wells with a pipettor (*see* **Note 6**).
8. Load 70 μL droplet generation oil into the bottom row of the cartridge ("Oil" row) (*see* **Note 8**).
9. Fit a gasket onto the cartridge.
10. Place cartridge into the droplet generator.
11. Remove the cartridge from the generator and use a multichannel pipettor to transfer droplets into a column of the 96-well PCR plate (*see* **Note 9**).
12. To generate droplets for the remaining samples, repeat **steps 3–10** (*see* **Note 10**).
13. Seal PCR plate with pierceable foil heat seal using a PCR plate sealer.
14. Run the PCR using the following program (*see* **Note 11**):

95 °C 10 min

40 cycles of

94 °C 30 s

60 °C 1 min

98 °C 10 min

4 °C hold

15. Read plate in the droplet reader according to the manufacturer's instruction and estimate the level of cross-sample contamination based on the number of events for the alternative allele (maximum value of all four SNPs). An example is shown in Fig. 2.

3.3 Detection of Contamination in Sequencing Data

1. Clone or download the Contamination Detection repository to your computer:

   git clone https://github.com/NWeinh/Contamination_Detection.git

2. For a single tumor/normal pair execute the Contamination Detection script:

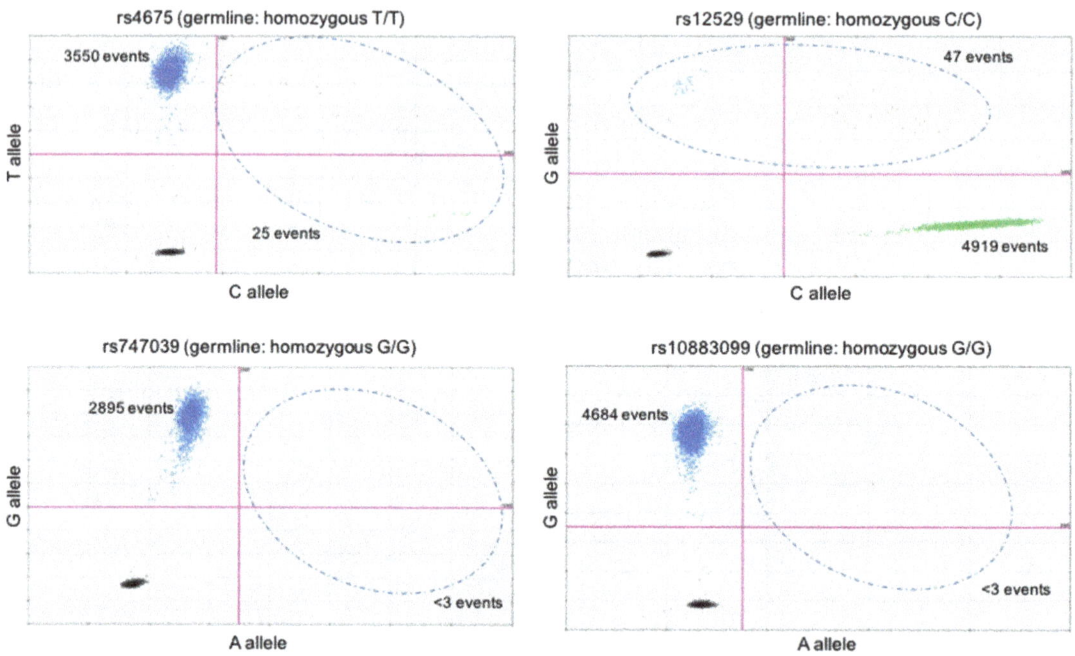

Fig. 2 Detection of cross-sample contamination. The figure shows the result of a ddPCR run for four SNPs of one tumor sample. For SNPs rs4675 and rs12529 25 (0.7% of total events) and 47 (0.9%) events indicate the alternative allele, respectively. For two SNPs (rs747039, rs10883099) less than three events for the alternative allele are detected (called negative, same genotype in contaminating sample). Thus, the tumor sample is contaminated and the estimated level of cross-sample contamination is 0.9% (maximum value of all four SNPs)

Rscript cont.R -t <TUMOR BAM> -g <GERMLINE BAM> -n <SAMPLE ID> -p <PATH TO contPanel.csv> -o <OUTFILE>

Note: For a list of all available command line options please consult the README of the github repository.

3. For multiple samples, modify file sampleSheet.csv and add sample IDs as well as location (full path) and name of tumor and control BAM files. One sample per row:

   SAMPLE_ID: patient identifier.

   CONTROL: BAM file name and location of the control (germ line) sample.

   TUMOR: BAM file name and location of the tumor sample.

   Then run:

   Rscript cont.R -s <SAMPLESHEET> -p <contPanel.csv> -o <OUTFILE>

4. The value in the "EstCont" column in the output file corresponds to the estimated level of cross-sample contamination in percent (*see* **Notes 12** and **13**). The script also calculates the background "noise," e.g., signals for C/T if the genotype is A/G. As such this tool can also be used to check the sequencing quality. An example for a patient with one contaminated and one noncontaminated tumor sample is shown in Table 2.

4 Notes

1. The contamination detection script was designed for the detection of contamination in whole exome and whole genome sequencing data. For application in targeted sequencing panels, please make sure that SNPs listed in contPanel.csv are included in the panel. As an alternative, you can provide your own set of control SNPs and adjust the contPanel.csv file accordingly.
2. We recommend a sequencing depth of 50× for control SNPs (default setting). The script will only use SNPs meeting this requirement.
3. The manufacturer's instruction can be downloaded at: https://www.fluidigm.com/binaries/content/documents/fluidigm/resources/flex-six-gt-taqman-fast-std-100-7719/flex-six-gt-taqman-fast-std-100-7719/fluidigm%3Afile.
4. Store unused 10× assay at −20 °C for up to 3 weeks.
5. According to our experience, four homozygous SNPs are sufficient for an initial screening of tumor samples. However, the sensitivity for detection of contaminated samples can be increased by analyzing more SNPs.

Table 2
Example output from contamination detection script

Sample	Patient_X_S1	Patient_X_S2	Patient_X_S3
Type	**Germ line**	**Tumor**	**Tumor**
N_Hom	113	113	113
NumSNP_Alt	1	94	5
NumSNP_A1	3	3	0
NumSNP_A2	1	4	4
Sum_Alt	1	754	6
Sum_A1	3	3	0
Sum_A2	1	5	4
Percent_Alt	0.88	83.19	4.4
Percent_A1	2.65	2.65	0
Percent_A2	0.88	3.54	3.5
PercentCont_Alt	0.007	4.66	0.02
PercentCont_A1	0.02	0.01	0
PercentCont_A2	0.006	0.02	0.02
Background	0.02	0.02	0.02
EstCont	0	9.28	0

N_Hom:** number of homozygous SNPs passing selection criteria; **NumSNP_Alt**: number of SNPs showing signals for the alternative allele; **NumSNP_A1/A2**: number of SNPs showing the third/fourth possible nucleotide, e.g., T or C if allele 1/2 are A/G; **Sum_: Corresponding total number of reads; **Percent_***: Percent of SNPs presenting the respective nucleotide; **PercentCont_***: Average proportion of reads showing respective nucleotide (calculated for "positive" SNPs only); **Background**: Maximum value of PercentCont_A1 and PercentCont_A2; EstCont: Estimate for cross-sample contamination. Corresponds to 2*(Percent_Cont_Alt—Background)

6. Avoid creating any bubbles, since this would reduce the droplet count in the generation step.
7. Pay attention to the orientation of the cartridge to ensure correct loading of samples to the 96-well PCR plate.
8. Oil should not be loaded before samples because this would reduce the droplet number.
9. Do not pipette too vigorously as this will shear the droplets.
10. To avoid cross contamination cover the PCR plate with the foil sheet while processing the remaining samples.
11. Do not exceed 50 PCR cycles.
12. Please be aware that the predicted level of contamination might be underestimated, e.g., if the sample is contaminated by more than one other sample. Importantly, cross-sample

contamination involving multiple samples from the same patient cannot be detected.

13. The sensitivity of this approach depends on the sequencing depth. We assume a sensitivity level of 1% at a depth of 100×.

Acknowledgement

This work was supported by the National Institute Of General Medical Sciences of the National Institutes of Health under Award Number P20GM125503. The content is solely the responsibility of the authors and does not necessarily represent the official views of the National Institutes of Health.

References

1. Rasche L, Chavan SS, Stephens OW, Patel PH, Tytarenko R, Ashby C et al (2017) Spatial genomic heterogeneity in multiple myeloma revealed by multi-region sequencing. Nat Commun 8:268
2. Bolli N, Avet-Loiseau H, Wedge DC, Van Loo P, Alexandrov LB, Martincorena I et al (2014) Heterogeneity of genomic evolution and mutational profiles in multiple myeloma. Nat Commun 5:2997
3. Lohr JG, Stojanov P, Carter SL, Cruz-Gordillo P, Lawrence MS, Auclair D et al (2014) Widespread genetic heterogeneity in multiple myeloma: implications for targeted therapy. Cancer Cell 25:91–101
4. Meißner T, Seckinger A, Rème T, Hielscher T, Möhler T, Neben K et al (2011) Gene expression profiling in multiple myeloma—reporting of entities, risk, and targets in clinical routine. Clin Cancer Res 17:7240–7247
5. Tirosh I, Izar B, Prakadan SM, Wadsworth MH 2nd, Treacy D, Trombetta JJ et al (2016) Dissecting the multicellular ecosystem of metastatic melanoma by single-cell RNA-seq. Science 352:189–196
6. Macosko EZ, Basu A, Satija R, Nemesh J, Shekhar K, Goldman M et al (2015) Highly parallel genome-wide expression profiling of individual cells using nanoliter droplets. Cell 161:1202–1214
7. Hu H, Liu X, Jin W, Hilger Ropers H, Wienker TF (2015) Evaluating information content of SNPs for sample-tagging in re-sequencing projects. Sci Rep 5:10247
8. Pengelly RJ, Gibson J, Andreoletti G, Collins A, Mattocks CJ, Ennis S (2013) A SNP profiling panel for sample tracking in whole-exome sequencing studies. Genome Med 5:89
9. Rajeevan H, Soundararajan U, Kidd JR, Pakstis AJ, Kidd KK (2012) ALFRED: an allele frequency resource for research and teaching. Nucleic Acids Res 40:D1010–D1015

Chapter 11

Analysis of Global Gene Expression Profiles

Alboukadel Kassambara and Jerome Moreaux

Abstract

DNA microarrays have considerably helped to improve the understanding of biological processes and diseases including multiple myeloma (MM). GEP analyses have been successful to classify MM, define risk, identify therapeutic targets, predict treatment response, and understand drug resistance.

This generated large amounts of publicly available data that could benefit from easy-to-use bioinformatics resources to analyze them. Here we present easy-to-use and open-access bioinformatics tools to extract and visualize the most prominent information from GEP data.

Key words Microarrays, Data mining, Bioinformatics, Multiple myeloma, GenomicScape, Molecular heterogeneity

1 Introduction

Genome-wide expression profile analysis with DNA microarrays has emerged as a powerful tool for biomedical research generating a huge amount of publicly available data. Microarrays have provided major inputs in the understanding of MM disease and important clinical applications [1–3]. In MM, GEP are used to classify the disease, define risk, identify therapeutic targets, predict treatment response, and understand drug resistance.

Microarray data provided new molecular classifications in MM underlying the heterogeneity of the disease [3–6]. Gene expression signatures associated with a poor outcome have been identified using microarrays and allow identification of patients with different disease course, which is useful to better rationalize treatment [2, 7–18]. Among these GEP-based risk signatures, several signatures were developed from direct identification of prognostic genes [7, 8, 12, 17] in newly diagnosed patients whereas other signatures related to biology were found to be of prognostic importance thereafter [9, 13–16, 18]. GEP approaches have also been used to study interactions between MM cells and the bone marrow microenvronment [19–25]. GEP has also been successfully used in MM

Christoph Heuck and Niels Weinhold (eds.), *Multiple Myeloma: Methods and Protocols*, Methods in Molecular Biology, vol. 1792, https://doi.org/10.1007/978-1-4939-7865-6_11,

to study drug response [26–31] or identify biomarkers associated with treatment sensitivity or resistance [10, 11, 27, 32–34].

These investigations generated a huge amount of publicly available GEP data. Although statistical programming frameworks like R and Bioconductor projects provide free bioinformatics packages to analyze the data, they remain difficult to use for untrained biologists or physicians, which limits the investigation of the large amounts of publicly available data. We provide here the description of easy-to-use and open access bioinformatics tools to extract and visualize the most prominent information from GEP data.

2 Materials

Based on our experience of mining high-throughput data to explore the biology of normal [35–39] and malignant plasma cells [1, 9–11, 14–16, 23, 40, 41], we have developed the current easy-to-use GenomicScape web tool (www.genomicscape.com) [39], which allows users to easily visualize and analyze gene expression data, and to explore the landscape of gene annotation resources for genes of interest (Fig. 1). Publicly available gene/ncRNA expression datasets from over 5000 microarray experiments performed on different cell types and obtained with Affymetrix, Illumina, or Agilent platforms have been uploaded into GenomicScape, which allows the user to readily extract information from these data. GenomicScape uses a MySQL database (version 5.1) for storing microarray data and gene annotations from usual databases (predominantly NCBI and Ensembl). The application core functionality, was developed with PHP version 5.3 utilizing R (http://www.r-project.org/) and Bioconductor (http://www.bioconductor.org/) scripts for data mining. The web interface is implemented with PHPBOOST web framework and uses jQWidgets javascript library.

Standard tools to mine microarray data have been implemented on GenomicScape. Briefly, the "Expression/Coexpression Report" tool allows the user to search for a gene using name or other identifiers, to visualize its expression profile in cell populations/tissues and to find genes whose expression in various samples are correlated to that of a given gene. The SAM tool uses the Significance Analysis of Microarrays (SAM) algorithms to identify genes differentially expressed between two groups (two-class paired or unpaired SAM analysis) or several groups (multiclass SAM analysis) of samples (http://statweb.stanford.edu/~tibs/SAM/).

To get a quick overview of the biological value of these genes, their expression and functional annotation can be visualized and exported by clicking their gene identifier. A heat map of the expression values of top-ranked genes across different sample groups can be generated and exported. The Principal Component Analysis

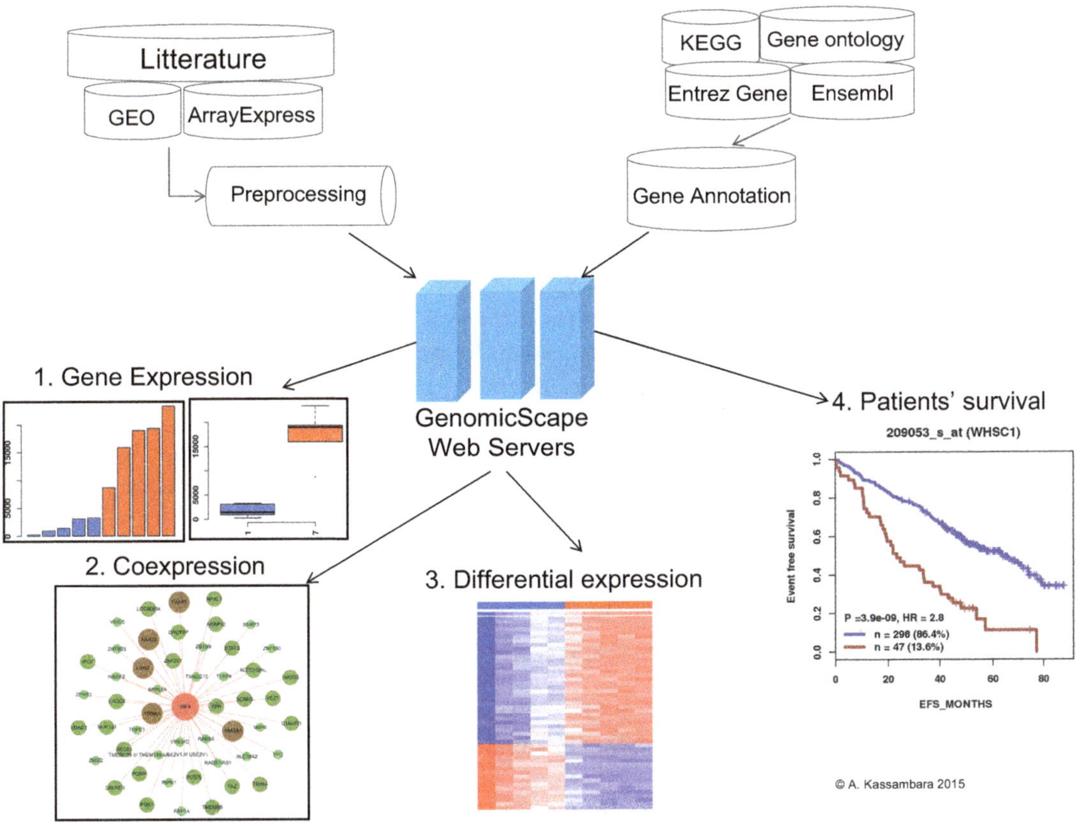

Fig. 1 Overview of GenomicScape webtools. The main tools, currently available on GenomicScape, are illustrated. GenomicScape allows users to (1) visualize the expression profile of one or multiple genes of interest in a given data set; (2) perform coexpression analysis; (3) analyze differentially expressed genes between cell subpopulations; and (4) to assess the link between a gene expression and patient's survival

(PCA) tool makes it possible to find how samples can group together using metric correlations, without making any assumption (unsupervised clustering). The PCA tool provides 2D and 3D visualizations of the samples plotted along the first 2–3 principal components. Sample colors are assigned by default or can be chosen by the user and tables and figures can be exported. The Survival Analysis tool allows the identification of genes associated with a prognostic value in different cohorts of patients.

3 Methods

3.1 Select a Dataset and Samples for Gene Expression Analyses

To select a dataset, click "Browse Data" in GenomicScape home page or use the following link: http://www.genomicscape.com/microarray/browsedata.php. More than 50 publicly available datasets comprising over 5000 microarray experiments have been presently uploaded into GenomicScape and can be used for analyses. These datasets include several cohorts of MM patients, normal bone marrow plasma cell samples, and human myeloma cell lines GEP data that have been organized according to the published biological experiments and the colors to visualize the gene expression in the groups preselected. The user may reorganize the samples, the groups, or the colors. Each group name is associated to a checkbox, which can be checked or unchecked to delete or add a given group in the analysis. By default, sample names are hidden. To choose the samples in a group, click "Show sample names" to display sample names and unselect or select samples. Several groups could also be merged to define new groups of samples. Once the groups and samples of interest have been selected, click "Analyze the data" at the bottom of the window. GenomicScape will display the tools to visualize or analyze the data. The tools Expression/coexpression Report, Significance of Analysis microarray, and Principal Component Analysis will be described.

3.2 Supervised Analysis to Compare Gene Expression Profiles of Different Cell Subpopulations

To load GenomicScape SAM tool, click "ANALYSIS TOOLS" and then "webSAM" from the home page or use the link: http://www.genomicscape.com/microarray/webSam.php.

- Choose a dataset and the sample groups to compare:
- The dataset "Arkansas, Myeloma (BMPC, MGUS, SMMC, MMC TT2)", used as example, is available under GenomicScape accession number GS-DT-48 (http://www.genomicscape.com/microarray/data_management.php?view=48).
- Samples and groups of the dataset are selected by default. The user can select the samples per group and the groups to compare as well as the colors assigned to each group for gene expression visualization (*see* Subheading 3.1).

Several filters are available to keep only genes of interest for GEP analyses. The first one makes it possible to keep only protein coding genes. The second one allows keeping only one probe set per gene/ncRNA according to the highest SD. Some probe sets interrogating identical gene, in particular those with a low signal, may provide unrelevant information, and could be deleted. The third one allows the selection of the number of probe sets with the highest SD. Indeed, a majority of probe sets has a low signal or is weakly differentially expressed between populations, which weakens the identification of interesting probe sets when applying multiple testing correction.

- Select filtering options of interest.
- Click "Apply" to move to the statistical test settings menu. To analyze the gene expression data with SAM tool, several parameters including Wilcoxon test, FDR (false discovery rate), fold change, number of permutation, and the type of

comparison (paired or unpaired) could be modified by the user. To compare GEP of purified MM cells from patients of the TT2 cohort (n = 345) with normal BMPC (n = 22), the parameters will be: Wilcoxon test, FDR ≤ 5%, Fold change ≥2, 1000 permutations and Unpaired test.

- Click "Submit." GenomicScape computes SAM algorithm and displays the genes differentially expressed between sample groups. The result is a list of genes ranked according to the SAM score, but can be ranked according to other SAM parameters. Clicking a gene name displays the expression of this gene in the various populations and its functional annotation.
- The name of sample groups used in the analysis is displayed at the bottom of the table. Clicking a group name displays the genes overexpressed in this group compared to the others.
- Below the gene table, several clickable buttons allow to export the gene set, analyze the gene set, or perform a heatmap of top genes.

3.3 Principal Component Analysis

- To load GenomicScape PCA tool, click "ANALYSIS TOOLS" and then "PRINCIPAL COMPONENT ANALYSIS" from the home page or use the following link: http://www.genomicscape.com/microarray/pca.php.
- Select the dataset and sample groups of interest as described above in the select dataset section. The user could paste a list of previously identified genes or select the number of genes with the highest variance between the samples to process PCA analysis. By default, the 2000 probe sets with the highest SD are kept for PCA, but this number can be modified. The user may also choose to get a movie of the 3D visualization of PCA. This option may reduce the speed of the computing.
- Click "Submit" to run the analysis.
- PCA output. GenomicScape provides the variance provided by each principal component and 2D and 3D visualizations of the samples plotted along the first 2–3 principal components. Colors are assigned to each sample according to its group belonging. The figures can be exported as PDF files. GenomicScape generates also a .txt file containing PCA results. This .txt file contains data including the coordinates of the samples and genes along principal component axes, which can be used to customize PCA plots.

3.4 Visualize Gene Expression Profile of a Set of Genes

- GenomicScape "Gene expression/Coexpression Report" tool allows the user to search for a gene by name or other identifiers, to visualize its expression profile in the populations of the selected dataset, and to find the genes correlated to a chosen gene. To use this tool, click "ANALYSIS TOOLS" and then

"EXPRESSION-COEXPRESSION REPORT" from GenomicScape home page or use the following link: http://www.genomicscape.com/microarray/expression.php.

- Select the dataset "Arkansas, Myeloma (BMPC, MGUS, SMMC, MMC TT2)".
- Select the groups and samples of interest as described above.
- Enter a list of genes or probe sets (one probe set per line and maximum number = 10,000).
- Clicking "Partial Match" or "Exact Match" indicates to look for genes whose name either contains the typed name or exactly matches with the typed name.
- Click "Submit."
- GenomicScape returns a clickable list of probe sets interrogating the genes of interest in the selected dataset. When several probe sets are available for a given gene, they are sorted from the highest to the lowest standard deviation (SD). A toolbar is available at the top of the search result to either "Plots all the genes" (i.e., visualize the expression of the probe set(s)) or "Export the gene set" or "Analyse the gene set."
- To get the probe sets coexpressed with a given probe set, click it. GenomicScape displays the gene expression plot of the clicked probe set in the selected populations as a barplot. Click "Coexpression Analysis" below the plot, choose the correlation parameters and then click "Submit." GenomicScape provides the list of genes correlated to the selected gene The heatmap and the coexpression network of the top correlated genes across selected populations are shown. From the coexpression network, the user may click a given coexpressed gene and GenomicScape will display the functional annotation and the coexpression plot of the gene.

3.5 Survival Analyses

Probe sets with prognostic significance can be identified using the Maxstat function [42] and the Benjamini–Hochberg multiple testing correction [16].

- GenomicScape "Survival Anlaysis" tool allows the user to search for a gene or a gene list by name or other identifiers and to investigate their prognostic value in cohorts of patients. To use this tool, click "ANALYSIS TOOLS" and then "SURVIVAL ANALYSIS" from GenomicScape home page or use the following link: http://www.genomicscape.com/microarray/survival.php.
- Select the dataset and sample groups of interest as described above in the select dataset section. The user could paste a list of previously identified genes and choose to run the analysis investigating overall survival (OS) or event free survival (EFS).

- Click "Submit" to run the analysis.
- Survival analysis output. GenomicScape provides the results of Maxstat analysis and survival curves are plotted using the Kaplan–Meier method for each tested gene. The statistical significance of differences in OS and EFS between patients' groups is calculated by using the log-rank test.
- GenomicScape returns a clickable list of probe sets interrogating the genes of interest in the selected dataset. When several probe sets are available for a given gene, they are sorted from the highest to the lowest standard deviation (SD). A toolbar is available at the top of the search result to either "Plots all the genes" (i.e., visualize the survival curves of the probe set(s)) or "Export the gene set" or "Analyse the gene set."
- The figures can be exported as PDF files. GenomicScape generates also a .txt file containing survival results. This .txt file contains data including the Maxstat cutpoint, p value, hazard ratio, and prognostic value of the investigated genes with expression levels or dichotomized values according to Maxstat algorithm. This .txt file could be used for Benjamini–Hochberg multiple testing correction in order to select the final list of prognostic genes.
- The prognostic value of these genes could be validated in an independent cohort of patients using the same approach.

3.6 Reactome and Gene Set Enrichment Analyses

The genes identified using SAM or Maxstat tools could be analyzed using Reactome or Gene Set Enrichment Analysis (GSEA) pathway enrichment tools [43, 44]. These tools allow to identify biological pathways significantly enriched among the identified genes differentially expressed between sample groups or associated with a significant prognostic value.

Gene set enrichment analysis is carried out by computing overlaps with canonical pathways and gene ontology gene sets obtained from Broad Institute (Cambridge, USA) (http://software.broadinstitute.org/gsea/index.jsp) [44]. The Reactome website (http://www.reactome.org) or Reactome Pathways Analysis R package (https://bioconductor.org/packages/release/bioc/html/ReactomePA.html) implement also enrichment analysis, gene set enrichment analysis and several functions for visualization [43].

Acknowledgments

This work was supported by grants from French INCA (Institut National du Cancer) Institute (PLBIO15-256) and ITMO Cancer (MM&TT).

References

1. Mahtouk K, Hose D, De Vos J, Moreaux J, Jourdan M, Rossi JF, Reme T, Goldschmidt H, Klein B (2007) Input of DNA microarrays to identify novel mechanisms in multiple myeloma biology and therapeutic applications. Clin Cancer Res 13(24):7289–7295
2. Chng WJ, Chung TH, Kumar S, Usmani S, Munshi N, Avet-Loiseau H, Goldschmidt H, Durie B, Sonneveld P (2016) Gene signature combinations improve prognostic stratification of multiple myeloma patients. Leukemia 30(5):1071–1078. https://doi.org/10.1038/leu.2015.341
3. Zhan F, Huang Y, Colla S, Stewart JP, Hanamura I, Gupta S, Epstein J, Yaccoby S, Sawyer J, Burington B, Anaissie E, Hollmig K, Pineda-Roman M, Tricot G, van Rhee F, Walker R, Zangari M, Crowley J, Barlogie B, Shaughnessy JD Jr (2006) The molecular classification of multiple myeloma. Blood 108(6):2020–2028. https://doi.org/10.1182/blood-2005-11-013458
4. Bergsagel PL, Kuehl WM, Zhan F, Sawyer J, Barlogie B, Shaughnessy J Jr (2005) Cyclin D dysregulation: an early and unifying pathogenic event in multiple myeloma. Blood 106(1):296–303. https://doi.org/10.1182/blood-2005-01-0034
5. Agnelli L, Bicciato S, Mattioli M, Fabris S, Intini D, Verdelli D, Baldini L, Morabito F, Callea V, Lombardi L, Neri A (2005) Molecular classification of multiple myeloma: a distinct transcriptional profile characterizes patients expressing CCND1 and negative for 14q32 translocations. J Clin Oncol 23(29):7296–7306. https://doi.org/10.1200/JCO.2005.01.3870
6. Zhou Y, Zhang Q, Stephens O, Heuck CJ, Tian E, Sawyer JR, Cartron-Mizeracki MA, Qu P, Keller J, Epstein J, Barlogie B, Shaughnessy JD Jr (2012) Prediction of cytogenetic abnormalities with gene expression profiles. Blood 119(21):e148–e150. https://doi.org/10.1182/blood-2011-10-388702
7. Reme T, Hose D, Theillet C, Klein B (2013) Modeling risk stratification in human cancer. Bioinformatics 29(9):1149–1157. https://doi.org/10.1093/bioinformatics/btt124
8. Shaughnessy JD Jr, Zhan F, Burington BE, Huang Y, Colla S, Hanamura I, Stewart JP, Kordsmeier B, Randolph C, Williams DR, Xiao Y, Xu H, Epstein J, Anaissie E, Krishna SG, Cottler-Fox M, Hollmig K, Mohiuddin A, Pineda-Roman M, Tricot G, van Rhee F, Sawyer J, Alsayed Y, Walker R, Zangari M, Crowley J, Barlogie B (2007) A validated gene expression model of high-risk multiple myeloma is defined by deregulated expression of genes mapping to chromosome 1. Blood 109(6):2276–2284. https://doi.org/10.1182/blood-2006-07-038430
9. Moreaux J, Klein B, Bataille R, Descamps G, Maiga S, Hose D, Goldschmidt H, Jauch A, Reme T, Jourdan M, Amiot M, Pellat-Deceunynck C (2011) A high-risk signature for patients with multiple myeloma established from the molecular classification of human myeloma cell lines. Haematologica 96(4):574–582. https://doi.org/10.3324/haematol.2010.033456
10. Moreaux J, Reme T, Leonard W, Veyrune JL, Requirand G, Goldschmidt H, Hose D, Klein B (2012) Development of gene expression-based score to predict sensitivity of multiple myeloma cells to DNA methylation inhibitors. Mol Cancer Ther 11(12):2685–2692. https://doi.org/10.1158/1535-7163.MCT-12-0721
11. Moreaux J, Reme T, Leonard W, Veyrune JL, Requirand G, Goldschmidt H, Hose D, Klein B (2013) Gene expression-based prediction of myeloma cell sensitivity to histone deacetylase inhibitors. Br J Cancer 109(3):676–685. https://doi.org/10.1038/bjc.2013.392
12. Decaux O, Lode L, Magrangeas F, Charbonnel C, Gouraud W, Jezequel P, Attal M, Harousseau JL, Moreau P, Bataille R, Campion L, Avet-Loiseau H, Minvielle S, Intergroupe Francophone du M (2008) Prediction of survival in multiple myeloma based on gene expression profiles reveals cell cycle and chromosomal instability signatures in high-risk patients and hyperdiploid signatures in low-risk patients: a study of the Intergroupe francophone du Myelome. J Clin Oncol Off J Am Soc Clin Oncol 26(29):4798–4805. https://doi.org/10.1200/JCO.2007.13.8545
13. Hose D, Reme T, Hielscher T, Moreaux J, Messner T, Seckinger A, Benner A, Shaughnessy JD Jr, Barlogie B, Zhou Y, Hillengass J, Bertsch U, Neben K, Mohler T, Rossi JF, Jauch A, Klein B, Goldschmidt H (2011) Proliferation is a central independent prognostic factor and target for personalized and risk-adapted treatment in multiple myeloma. Haematologica 96(1):87–95. https://doi.org/10.3324/haematol.2010.030296
14. Kassambara A, Gourzones-Dmitriev C, Sahota S, Reme T, Moreaux J, Goldschmidt H, Constantinou A, Pasero P, Hose D, Klein B (2014) A DNA repair pathway score predicts survival in human multiple myeloma: the potential for therapeutic strategy. Oncotarget 5(9):2487–2498

15. Kassambara A, Hose D, Moreaux J, Reme T, Torrent J, Rossi JF, Goldschmidt H, Klein B (2012) Identification of pluripotent and adult stem cell genes unrelated to cell cycle and associated with poor prognosis in multiple myeloma. PLoS One 7(7):e42161. https://doi.org/10.1371/journal.pone.0042161

16. Kassambara A, Hose D, Moreaux J, Walker BA, Protopopov A, Reme T, Pellestor F, Pantesco V, Jauch A, Morgan G, Goldschmidt H, Klein B (2012) Genes with a spike expression are clustered in chromosome (sub)bands and spike (sub)bands have a powerful prognostic value in patients with multiple myeloma. Haematologica 97(4):622–630. https://doi.org/10.3324/haematol.2011.046821

17. Kuiper R, Broyl A, de Knegt Y, van Vliet MH, van Beers EH, van der Holt B, el Jarari L, Mulligan G, Gregory W, Morgan G, Goldschmidt H, Lokhorst HM, van Duin M, Sonneveld P (2012) A gene expression signature for high-risk multiple myeloma. Leukemia 26(11):2406–2413. https://doi.org/10.1038/leu.2012.127

18. Chng WJ, Braggio E, Mulligan G, Bryant B, Remstein E, Valdez R, Dogan A, Fonseca R (2008) The centrosome index is a powerful prognostic marker in myeloma and identifies a cohort of patients that might benefit from aurora kinase inhibition. Blood 111(3):1603–1609. https://doi.org/10.1182/blood-2007-06-097774

19. Corre J, Mahtouk K, Attal M, Gadelorge M, Huynh A, Fleury-Cappellesso S, Danho C, Laharrague P, Klein B, Reme T, Bourin P (2007) Bone marrow mesenchymal stem cells are abnormal in multiple myeloma. Leukemia 21(5):1079–1088

20. Moreaux J, Hose D, Kassambara A, Reme T, Moine P, Requirand G, Goldschmidt H, Klein B (2011) Osteoclast-gene expression profiling reveals osteoclast-derived CCR2 chemokines promoting myeloma cell migration. Blood 117(4):1280–1290. https://doi.org/10.1182/blood-2010-04-279760

21. Vacca A, Scavelli C, Montefusco V, Di Pietro G, Neri A, Mattioli M, Bicciato S, Nico B, Ribatti D, Dammacco F, Corradini P (2005) Thalidomide downregulates angiogenic genes in bone marrow endothelial cells of patients with active multiple myeloma. J Clin Oncol 23(23):5334–5346

22. Hose D, Moreaux J, Meissner T, Seckinger A, Goldschmidt H, Benner A, Mahtouk K, Hillengass J, Reme T, De Vos J, Hundemer M, Condomines M, Bertsch U, Rossi JF, Jauch A, Klein B, Mohler T (2009) Induction of angiogenesis by normal and malignant plasma cells. Blood 114(1):128–143. https://doi.org/10.1182/blood-2008-10-184226

23. Mahtouk K, Moreaux J, Hose D, Reme T, Meissner T, Jourdan M, Rossi JF, Pals ST, Goldschmidt H, Klein B (2010) Growth factors in multiple myeloma: a comprehensive analysis of their expression in tumor cells and bone marrow environment using Affymetrix microarrays. BMC Cancer 10:198. https://doi.org/10.1186/1471-2407-10-198

24. Moreaux J, Cremer FW, Reme T, Raab M, Mahtouk K, Kaukel P, Pantesco V, De Vos J, Jourdan E, Jauch A, Legouffe E, Moos M, Fiol G, Goldschmidt H, Rossi JF, Hose D, Klein B (2005) The level of TACI gene expression in myeloma cells is associated with a signature of microenvironment dependence versus a plasmablastic signature. Blood 106(3):1021–1030

25. Moreaux J, Legouffe E, Jourdan E, Quittet P, Reme T, Lugagne C, Moine P, Rossi JF, Klein B, Tarte K (2004) BAFF and APRIL protect myeloma cells from apoptosis induced by interleukin 6 deprivation and dexamethasone. Blood 103(8):3148–3157

26. Burington B, Barlogie B, Zhan F, Crowley J, Shaughnessy JD Jr (2008) Tumor cell gene expression changes following short-term in vivo exposure to single agent chemotherapeutics are related to survival in multiple myeloma. Clin Cancer Res 14(15):4821–4829. https://doi.org/10.1158/1078-0432.CCR-07-4568

27. Shaughnessy JD Jr, Qu P, Usmani S, Heuck CJ, Zhang Q, Zhou Y, Tian E, Hanamura I, van Rhee F, Anaissie E, Epstein J, Nair B, Stephens O, Williams R, Waheed S, Alsayed Y, Crowley J, Barlogie B (2011) Pharmacogenomics of bortezomib test-dosing identifies hyperexpression of proteasome genes, especially PSMD4, as novel high-risk feature in myeloma treated with Total therapy 3. Blood 118(13):3512–3524. https://doi.org/10.1182/blood-2010-12-328252

28. Mulligan G, Mitsiades C, Bryant B, Zhan F, Chng WJ, Roels S, Koenig E, Fergus A, Huang Y, Richardson P, Trepicchio WL, Broyl A, Sonneveld P, Shaughnessy JD Jr, Bergsagel PL, Schenkein D, Esseltine DL, Boral A, Anderson KC (2007) Gene expression profiling and correlation with outcome in clinical trials of the proteasome inhibitor bortezomib. Blood 109(8):3177–3188. https://doi.org/10.1182/blood-2006-09-044974

29. Neri P, Tagliaferri P, Di Martino MT, Calimeri T, Amodio N, Bulotta A, Ventura M, Eramo PO, Viscomi C, Arbitrio M, Rossi M, Caraglia M, Munshi NC, Anderson KC, Tassone P (2008) In vivo anti-myeloma activity and mod-

ulation of gene expression profile induced by valproic acid, a histone deacetylase inhibitor. Br J Haematol 143(4):520–531. https://doi.org/10.1111/j.1365-2141.2008.07387.x

30. Chauhan D, Auclair D, Robinson EK, Hideshima T, Li G, Podar K, Gupta D, Richardson P, Schlossman RL, Krett N, Chen LB, Munshi NC, Anderson KC (2002) Identification of genes regulated by dexamethasone in multiple myeloma cells using oligonucleotide arrays. Oncogene 21(9):1346–1358
31. Mitsiades CS, Mitsiades NS, McMullan CJ, Poulaki V, Shringarpure R, Hideshima T, Akiyama M, Chauhan D, Munshi N, Gu X, Bailey C, Joseph M, Libermann TA, Richon VM, Marks PA, Anderson KC (2004) Transcriptional signature of histone deacetylase inhibition in multiple myeloma: biological and clinical implications. Proc Natl Acad Sci U S A 101(2):540–545
32. Maes K, De Smedt E, Kassambara A, Hose D, Seckinger A, Van Valckenborgh E, Menu E, Klein B, Vanderkerken K, Moreaux J, De Bruyne E (2015) In vivo treatment with epigenetic modulating agents induces transcriptional alterations associated with prognosis and immunomodulation in multiple myeloma. Oncotarget 6(5):3319–3334
33. Kronke J, Kuchenbauer F, Kull M, Teleanu V, Bullinger L, Bunjes D, Greiner A, Kolmus S, Kopff S, Schreder M, Mugge LO, Straka C, Engelhardt M, Dohner H, Einsele H, Bassermann F, Bargou R, Knop S, Langer C (2017) IKZF1 expression is a prognostic marker in newly diagnosed standard-risk multiple myeloma treated with lenalidomide and intensive chemotherapy: a study of the German myeloma study group (DSMM). Leukemia 31(6):1363–1367. https://doi.org/10.1038/leu.2016.384
34. Bila J, Sretenovic A, Jelicic J, Tosic N, Glumac I, Fekete MD, Antic D, Balint MT, Markovic O, Milojevic Z, Radojkovic M, Trajkovic G, Puric M, Pavlovic S, Mihaljevic B (2016) Prognostic significance of Cereblon expression in patients with multiple myeloma. Clin Lymphoma Myeloma Leuk 16(11):610–615. https://doi.org/10.1016/j.clml.2016.08.007
35. Jourdan M, Caraux A, Caron G, Robert N, Fiol G, Reme T, Bollore K, Vendrell JP, Le Gallou S, Mourcin F, De Vos J, Kassambara A, Duperray C, Hose D, Fest T, Tarte K, Klein B (2011) Characterization of a transitional preplasmablast population in the process of human B cell to plasma cell differentiation. J Immunol 187(8):3931–3941. https://doi.org/10.4049/jimmunol.1101230
36. Jourdan M, Caraux A, De Vos J, Fiol G, Larroque M, Cognot C, Bret C, Duperray C, Hose D, Klein B (2009) An in vitro model of differentiation of memory B cells into plasmablasts and plasma cells including detailed phenotypic and molecular characterization. Blood 114(25):5173–5181. https://doi.org/10.1182/blood-2009-07-235960
37. Jourdan M, Cren M, Robert N, Bollore K, Fest T, Duperray C, Guilloton F, Hose D, Tarte K, Klein B (2014) IL-6 supports the generation of human long-lived plasma cells in combination with either APRIL or stromal cell-soluble factors. Leukemia 28(8):1647–1656. https://doi.org/10.1038/leu.2014.61
38. Schoenhals M, Jourdan M, Seckinger A, Pantesco V, Hose D, Kassambara A, Moreaux J, Klein B (2016) Forced KLF4 expression increases the generation of mature plasma cells and uncovers a network linked with plasma cell stage. Cell Cycle 15(14):1919–1928. https://doi.org/10.1080/15384101.2016.1191709
39. Kassambara A, Reme T, Jourdan M, Fest T, Hose D, Tarte K, Klein B (2015) GenomicScape: an easy-to-use web tool for gene expression data analysis. Application to investigate the molecular events in the differentiation of B cells into plasma cells. PLoS Comput Biol 11(1):e1004077. https://doi.org/10.1371/journal.pcbi.1004077
40. Viziteu E, Grandmougin C, Goldschmidt H, Seckinger A, Hose D, Klein B, Moreaux J (2016) Chetomin, targeting HIF-1alpha/p300 complex, exhibits antitumour activity in multiple myeloma. Br J Cancer 114(5):519–523. https://doi.org/10.1038/bjc.2016.20
41. Viziteu E, Klein B, Basbous J, Lin YL, Hirtz C, Gourzones C, Tiers L, Bruyer A, Vincent L, Grandmougin C, Seckinger A, Goldschmidt H, Constantinou A, Pasero P, Hose D, Moreaux J (2017) RECQ1 helicase is involved in replication stress survival and drug resistance in multiple myeloma. Leukemia 31(10):2104–2113. https://doi.org/10.1038/leu.2017.54
42. Hothorn T, Lausen B (2003) On the exact distribution of maximally selected rank statistics. Comput Stat Data Anal 43(2):121–137. https://doi.org/10.1016/S0167-9473(02)00225-6
43. Yu G, He QY (2016) ReactomePA: an R/bioconductor package for reactome pathway analysis and visualization. Mol BioSyst 12(2):477–479. https://doi.org/10.1039/c5mb00663e
44. Subramanian A, Tamayo P, Mootha VK, Mukherjee S, Ebert BL, Gillette MA, Paulovich A, Pomeroy SL, Golub TR, Lander ES, Mesirov JP (2005) Gene set enrichment analysis: a knowledge-based approach for interpreting genome-wide expression profiles. Proc Natl Acad Sci U S A 102(43):15545–15550. https://doi.org/10.1073/pnas.0506580102

Chapter 12

Genome Wide Mapping of Methylated and Hydroxyl-Methylated Cytosines Using a Modified HpaII Tiny Fragment Enrichment by Ligation Mediated PCR Tagged Sequencing Protocol

Sanchari Battachariyya, Ruslana Tytarenko, Christoph Heuck, John Greally, and Amit Verma

Abstract

Here we describe a method for genome wide investigation of methylation and hydroxymethylation status of cytosines. This protocol is an improvement of the HELP-tagging protocol previously described by Suzuki et al. It involves the glucosylation of 5-hydroxymethylcytosines (5-hmC) with β-glucosyl transferase (β-GT), thus rendering them resistant to digestion by MspI. Parallel digestion of β-GT treated samples with MspI, untreated sample with MspI and another untreated sample with HpaII, followed by adapter ligation, parallel sequencing and bioinformatics processing results in a differential display of MspI digestion sites that allows the determination of the distribution of 5-methylcytosines (5-mC) and 5-hmC at these sites.

Key words 5-methylcytosine, 5-hydroxymethylcytosine, Sequencing, β-glucosyl transferase, HpaII, MspI, DNA methylation

1 Introduction

Epigenetic mechanisms can influence gene expression. They are involved in cell differentiation but can also have deleterious effects that can result in malignant transformation of the cells. Genome wide DNA methylation studies in MM have revealed stage specific changes and association with outcome [1, 2]. The role of epigenetic factors in myeloma genesis and the opportunities for therapeutic intervention have recently been reviewed by Alzrigat et al. [3]. The most widely studied epigenetic mechanism is DNA methylation. It involves the covalent binding of a methyl group to cytosine at the carbon 5 position (5-mC) in the context of CpG dinucleotides. The pattern of DNA methylation controls chromatin structure, target sites for DNA binding proteins and ultimately affects gene expression [4].

Christoph Heuck and Niels Weinhold (eds.), *Multiple Myeloma: Methods and Protocols*, Methods in Molecular Biology, vol. 1792, https://doi.org/10.1007/978-1-4939-7865-6_12,

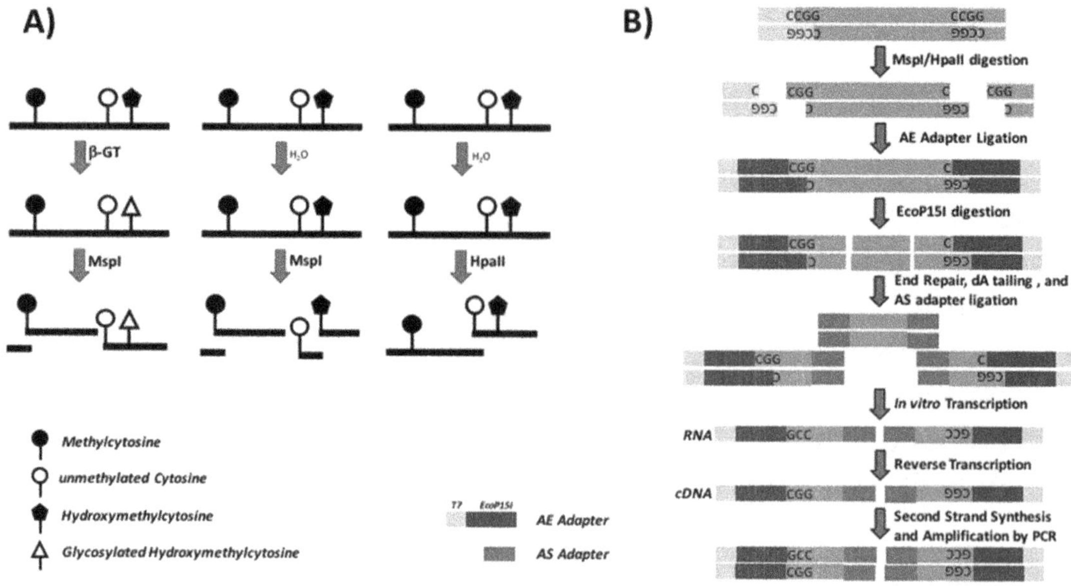

Fig. 1 Schematic summary of the HELP-GT assay (adapted from Bhattacharyya et al. [8]). (**a**) Genomic DNA with Hpa II (right panel), MspI (middle panel), or MspI after β-GT pretreatment (left panel). HpaII only cuts at CCGG sequences where the central CCGG dinucleotide is unmethylated. MspI digests regardless of methylation context. Pretreatment with β-GT renders CCGG sequences, where the central C is hydroxymethylated insensitive to MSPI digestion. (**b**) The first Illumina adapter (AE) is ligated to the cohesive end created by the digestion, juxtaposing an EcoP15I site beside the HpaII/MspI digestion site and allowing EcoP15I to digest within the flanking DNA sequence as shown. An A overhang is created, allowing the ligation of the second Illumina adapter (AS). A T7 polymerase-mediated in vitro transcription from a promoter sequence located on the AE adapter, selectively enriches for the AE-insert-AS products. A limited PCR amplification generates a single-sized product for Illumina sequencing. The final library can be sequenced on Illumina HiSeq2000 (50 bp single end reads) using a custom sequencing primer

DNA methylation is an active process mediated by DNA methyl transferases. For a long time reversal of this DNA methylation was seen as a passive process, either through spontaneous deamination or loss of the methylation marks during DNA replication. More recently DNA hydroxymethylation has been proposed as a specific intermediate in the active demethylation pathway. In particular, TET proteins have been shown to mediate the active dioxygenation of 5-mC to 5-hydroxymethyl cytosine (5-hmC) [5]. The discovery of mutations of IDH and TET proteins in various hematologic neoplasms also suggests that defects in 5-hmC pathway have functional consequences in carcinogenesis [6, 7].

The HELP-GT assay [8] described below is based on the HpaII tiny fragment Enrichment by Ligation-mediated PCR (HELP) assay originally published by Kuhlan et al. [9] and its adaptations for massive parallel sequencing, the HELP tagging assay [10]. In brief, the HELP assay takes advantage of the isoschizomers HpaII and MspI which both recognize the and cut the CCGG motive (Fig. 1). HpaII is methylation sensitive and will only digest CCGGs where the central C is unmethylated. In contrast MspI is methylation insensitive in will digest CCGGs irrespective of methylation status. Similarly CCGGs with hydroxymethylated central Cs will be digested by MspI whereas HpaII will leave these sequences untouched thus making 5mCs and 5hmC indistinguishable using the standard HELP method. Glycosylation of 5hmCs using beta glucosyl transferase (β-GT) renders those sites insensitive to digestions with MspI. The HELP-GT assay uses three parallel restriction digests, with HpaII, MspI, and MspI after β-GT conversion, respectively followed by adapter ligation and massive parallel sequencing to accurately quantify the methylation and hydroxymethylation status at >1.3 million HpaII digestion sites throughout the human genome.

2 Materials

2.1 Reagents (see Note 1)

T4 Phage β-glucosyltransferase (T4-BGT)	NEB
Agarose	
TAE buffer (50×)	Bio rad #161–0743
Glycogen	
Isopropanol	
dNTP nucleotides (100 mM)	Invitrogen
HpaII	NEB
MspI	NEB
EcoP15I	NEB
Phusion high Fidelity DNA polymerase	NEB
Klenow fragment (3'→5' exo-)	NEB
Quick ligation kit	NEB
T4 DNA polymerase	NEB
T4 DNA polynucleotide kinase	NEB
T4 DNA ligase buffer	NEB
MEGAshortscript kit	Ambion
SuperscriptIII reverse transcription kit	Invitrogen
DIUF water	
QiaQuick PCR purification kit	Qiagen
MinElute PCR purification kit	Qiagen
RNeasy clean up kit MinElute	Qiagen
AMPure XP 5 ml kit	Agencourt

TE buffer, pH 8	Add 10 mL of 1 M Tris–HCl (pH 8) and 1 mL of 1 M EDTA and fill up to 1 L with DIUF water; autoclave
Ethachinmate	Wako
QiaQuick gel extraction kit	Qiagen

2.1.1 Equipment

PCR thermal cycler

Gel system and power source

Water bath

Benchtop microcentrifuge

PCR plate magnet (e.g., SPRIPlate 96R; Agencourt #A29164)

2.1.2 Primer Sequences and Preparation

Adapter sequence (Solexa end)

AS_1: 5′-ACACTCTTTCCCTACACGACGCTCTTCCGATC-x-T (x: phosphorothioate bond)

AS_2: 5′-p-GATCGGAAGAGCGTCGTGTAGGGAAAGAGTGT

Adapter sequences (EcoP15I end)

AE_1: 5′-ACAGTAATACGACTCACTATAGGGAGAAGGCTCAAGCAGAAGACGGCATACGACAGCAG

AE_2: 5′-p-CGCTGCTGTCGTATGCCGTCTTCTGCTTGAGCCTTCTCCCTATAGTGAGTCGTATTACTG*T

(*T: inverted dT)

PCR primer

PS: 5′-AATGATACGGCGACCACCGAGATCTACACTCTTTCCCTACACGACGCTCTTCCGATCT

PE: 5′-CAAGCAGAAGACGGCATACGACAGCAG

Sequencing primer

PSeq: 5′-ACACTCTTTCCCTACACGACGCTCTTCCGATCT

Set up AS annealing reaction in a PCR tube as follows:

Primer AS_1 (100 μM)	20 μL
Primer AS_2 (100 μM)	20 μL
TE	10 μL
Total	50 μL

Place primer mix in a thermal cycler at 97.5 °C for 150 s and then ramping down to 4 °C over the course of 1 h. The final concentration of the AS primer stock will be 40 μM.

Set up AS annealing reaction in a PCR tube as follows:

Primer AE_1 (100 μM)	20 μL
Primer AE_2 (100 μM)	20 μL
TE	10 μL
Total	50 μL

Place primer mix in a thermal cycler at 97.5 °C for 150 s and then ramping down to 4 °C over the course of 1 h. The final concentration of the AS primer stock will be 40 μM.

3 Method

1. Set up 2 PCR tubes per digestion as follows (total of 6 tubes). Incubate 9–16 h at 37 °C.

	MspI digest	**MspI digest + βGT**	**HpaII digest**
Genomic DNA	200 ng	200 ng	200 ng
10× NEB buffer 4	10 μL	10 μL	–
10× NEB buffer 1	–	–	10 μL
2 mM UDPG (50×)	4 μL	4 μL	4 μL
T4 β GT	–	3 μL	–
DIUF water	To final 100 μL total	To final 100 μL total	To final 100 μL total

Remove 3 μL from each tube and save for quality control in **step 3** below.

2. Add enzymes for digestions to tubes from **step 1** as follows:

	MspI digest	**MspI digest + βGT**	**HpaII digest**
MspI	3 μL	3 μl	–
HpaII	–	–	3 μl

Incubate 16 h at 37 °C.

3. Remove 3 μL from each tube. Run all samples of the digest and the samples saved from **step 1** above on 1% agarose gel. Samples from **step 1** will serve as a "undigested control" for samples from **step 2**.You should be able to see the difference between the two digests. With HpaII most of the DNA remains

high molecular weight, whereas with the MspI digest there should be an almost even smear with almost no high molecular weight DNA.

4. Digest purification with the Gentra Puregene kit (*see* **Note 2**):
   (a) Add 80 μL of lysis buffer (Gentra Puregene kit) to the digestion reaction. Vortex and quickly spin down.
   (b) Add 60 μL of protein precipitation solution, vortex, incubate on ice for 15 min. Centrifuge for 3 min.
   (c) Carefully collect the supernatant and transfer to a new clean 1.5 mL tube with 200 μL of isopropanol (molecular grade) plus 1 μL of Ethachinmate.
   (d) Precipitate DNA by inverting tube 10 times.
   (e) Incubate for 30 min at −20 °C. Centrifuge for 15 min.
   (f) Carefully discard the supernatant.
   (g) Wash pellet with freshly prepared 70% Ethanol.
   (h) Resuspend pellet in 6 μL PCR grade water.
5. Set up AE ligation in a PCR tube as follows:

2× Quick ligase buffer	6.5 μL
DNA from last step	5 μL
Adapter AE (0.1 μM mix)	0.5 μL
Quick ligase	1 μL
Total	13 μL

   Incubate at room temperature for 15 min.
6. After AE ligation, purify the products with AMpure and elute with 19.75 μL of nuclease free water.
7. Set up the EcoP15I digestion as follows in a PCR tube.

Purified ligation mix from last step	18.25 μL
NEB buffer 3(10×)	2.5 μL
ATP (10×)	2.5 μL
BSA (100×)	0.25 μL
EcoP15I	1.5 μL
Total	25 μL

   Incubate at 37 °C overnight.
8. After EcoP15I digestion purify the digested product with QIAquick PCR purification kit. Elute with 21 μL of EB buffer (*see* **Note 3**).

9. Set up end repair reaction as follows:

DNA from last step	19.5 μL
T4 DNA ligase buffer with ATP (10×)	2.5 μL
dNTP (10 mM)	0.5 μL
T4 DNA polymerase	1.25 μL
T4 DNA polynucleotide kinase	1.25 μL
Total	25 μL

Incubate at 37 °C for 30 min

10. After end repair, purify the products with QIAquick mini elute PCR purification kit. Elute with 20.5 μL of EB buffer (*see* **Note 3**).
11. Set up dA tailing reaction in a PCR tube as follows:

DNA from last step	19 μL
NEB buffer 2 (10×)	3 μL
Klenow (3′ ≥ 5′ exo)	1.5 μL
dATP (1 μM)	5 μL
DIUF water	1.5 μL
Total	30 μL

Incubate at 37 °C for 30 min.

12. After dA tailing reaction, purify the products with QIAquick mini elute PCR purification kit. Elute with 14.5 μL of EB buffer (also *see* **Note 3**).
13. Set up AS ligation reaction in a PCR tube as follows: (barcoded AS primers used here if desired).

DNA from last step	12.5 μL
2× quick ligase buffer	15 μL
Adapter AS (1 μM)	1 μL
Quick ligase	1.5 μL
Total	30 μL

Incubate at room temperature for 15 min.

14. After AS ligation purify the products with MinElute PCR purification kit. Elute with 10 μL of EB buffer (also *see* **Note 3**).
15. Set up in vitro transcription with MEGA shortscript kit in a PCR tube as follows

DNA from last step	8 μL
T7 10× reaction buffer	2 μL
T7 ATP solution (75 mM)	2 μL

T7 CTP solution (75 mM)	2 μL
T7 GTP solution (75 mM)	2 μL
T7 UTP solution (75 mM)	2 μL
T7 enzyme mix	2 μL
Total	20 μL

Incubate at 37 °C for 16 h.
Add to same tube.

DNAse TURBO	1 μL
Total	21 μL

Incubate at 37 °C for 15 min.

16. After in vitro transcription purify the product with RNeasy clean-up kit MinElute and elute with 10 μL of RNAse free water (*see* **Note 3**).
17. Set up RT reaction with SuperScript III reverse transcription kit in a PCR tube as follows:

RNA from last setup	8 μL
Primer (PS) 2 μM	1 μL
dNTPs	1 μL
Total	10 μL

Incubate at 65 °C for 5 min and chill on ice.
Add to the same tube.

10× RT buffer	2 μL
0.1 M DTT	2 μL
MgCl2	4 μL
RNAse out	1 μL
SuperScript III	1 μL
Total	20 μL

Incubate at 25 °C for 5 min, followed by 50 °C for 60 min, followed by 80 °C for 10 min.
Add to the same tube.

RNAse H	1 μL
Total	21 μL

Incubate at 37 ° C for 20 min.

18. RT purification with Gentra Puregene Kit (*see* **Note 4**):
    (a) Add 40uL of lysis buffer RT product from previous step.

(b) Add 20uL of protein precipitation solution, vortex, incubate on ice for 5 min, spin for 5 min, and collect supernatant.

(c) Add 60uL of isopropanol and 0.5uL of ethachinmate to new tube, and mix with supernatant, mix by inverting the tube for 10 times, incubate for 30 min at −20 °C.

(d) Spin for 15 min.

(e) Remove supernatant and wash pellet with 70% ethanol.

(f) Air-dry pellet and resuspend in 20 μL of DIUF water.

19. Set up PCR reaction with Superscript reverse transcription kit in a PCR tube as follows:
Set up two tubes for each digest (*see* also **Note 5**).

RT product from previous step	10 μL
5× HF buffer	10 μL
Primer PS (10 μM)	0.5 μL
Primer PE (10 μM)	0.5 μL
dNTP mix (10 mM)	1 μL
DIUF water	27.5 μL
Phusion polymerase	0.5 μL
Total	50 μL

Cycle as follows:

2 min at 98 °C

18 cycles of

15 s at 98 °C

15 s at 60 °C

15 s at 72 °C

Followed by

2 min at 72 °C

Hold at 4 °C

20. Check product on a 3% agarose gel using a 20 bp ladder. Expect a product of 120 bp length.

21. Clean the product using a QIAGEN gel extraction kit. Elute with 30–40 μL of EB buffer.

Sequencing

22. Hybridize to Illumina flow cell at approximately 8pM according to manufacturer's protocol

4 Notes

1. To assure quality of the reagents limit the number of freeze-thaw cycles for the stock solutions
2. Alternative method the phenol and chloroform method maybe used:
   (a) Add 400 μL o TE buffer (pH 8.0) and 500 mL of saturated phenol–chloroform mix (1:1) and mix well. Centrifuge at top speed in a microcentrifuge for 10 min.
   (b) Take aqueous phase (about 500 μL) from last step, put into new tube and add 1 μL of glycogen and 50 μL of 3 M sodium acetate and mix well. Then add 800 μL of isopropanol, vortex and incubate at −20 °C for 30 min and centrifuge at top speed for 20 min.
   (c) Remove the supernatant and wash the pellet with 70% ethanol and air-dry. Once the pellet is air-dry, resuspend the pellet in 6 μL of TE. Measure the concentration with the NanoDrop spectrophotometer.
   (d) Proceed to AE ligation step.
3. Make sure that there is no remaining liquid in the column before loading the EB buffer. Since elution is performed with small volumes of EB buffer, carryover of small amounts of wash buffer may affect the following step.
4. In our hands the most efficient way to purify the RT product is by using the Gentra Puregene Kit. If this kit is not available you can use the following alternative procedure for RT product purification:

RT product from previous step	21 μL
DIUF water	80 μL
Ammonium acetate	50 μL
Ethachinmate (or glycogen)	1 μL
Ethanol (100%)	300 μL

   Mix and keep at −20 °C for 2 h.

   Centrifuge at full speed for 30 min.

   Remove supernatant.

   Wash twice with 70% ethanol (spin at full speed 2–3 min each time).
5. To reduce PCR bias, perform 3 PCRs and combine them in one tube afterwards.

References

1. Heuck CJ, Mehta J, Bhagat T et al (2013) Myeloma is characterized by stage-specific alterations in DNA methylation that occur early during myelomagenesis. J Immunol 190:2966–2975. https://doi.org/10.4049/jimmunol.1202493
2. Walker BA, Wardell CP, Chiecchio L et al (2011) Aberrant global methylation patterns affect the molecular pathogenesis and prognosis of multiple myeloma. Blood 117:553–562. https://doi.org/10.1182/blood-2010-04-279539
3. Alzrigat M, Párraga AA, Jernberg-Wiklund H (2017) Epigenetics in multiple myeloma: from mechanisms to therapy. Semin Cancer Biol. https://doi.org/10.1016/j.semcancer.2017.09.007
4. Brena RM, Huang TH-M, Plass C (2006) Toward a human epigenome. Nat Genet 38:1359–1360. https://doi.org/10.1038/ng1206-1359
5. Tahiliani M, Koh KP, Shen Y et al (2009) Conversion of 5-methylcytosine to 5-hydroxymethylcytosine in mammalian DNA by MLL partner TET1. Science 324:930–935. https://doi.org/10.1126/science.1170116
6. Abdel-Wahab O, Mullally A, Hedvat C et al (2009) Genetic characterization of TET1, TET2, and TET3 alterations in myeloid malignancies. Blood 114:144–147. https://doi.org/10.1182/blood-2009-03-210039
7. Figueroa ME, Abdel-Wahab O, Lu C et al (2010) Leukemic IDH1 and IDH2 mutations result in a hypermethylation phenotype, disrupt TET2 function, and impair hematopoietic differentiation. Cancer Cell 18:553–567. https://doi.org/10.1016/j.ccr.2010.11.015
8. Bhattacharyya S, Yu Y, Suzuki M et al (2013) Genome-wide hydroxymethylation tested using the HELP-GT assay shows redistribution in cancer. Nucleic Acids Res 41:e157. https://doi.org/10.1093/nar/gkt601
9. Khulan B, Thompson RF, Ye K et al (2006) Comparative isoschizomer profiling of cytosine methylation: the HELP assay. Genome Res 16:1046–1055. https://doi.org/10.1101/gr.5273806
10. Suzuki M, Jing Q, Lia D et al (2010) Optimized design and data analysis of tag-based cytosine methylation assays. Genome Biol 11:R36. https://doi.org/10.1186/gb-2010-11-4-r36

Chapter 13

A Rapid and Robust Protocol for Reduced Representation Bisulfite Sequencing in Multiple Myeloma

Samrat Roy Choudhury and Brian A. Walker

Abstract

Reduced representation bisulfite sequencing (RRBS) is one of the most comprehensive yet economic ways of mapping whole genome DNA-methylation. Here, we have substantially modified the RRBS protocol by combining end-repair and A-tailing steps, and by introducing a bead-based method for rapid and easy size selection of the library molecules. The method has been optimized for myeloma clinical samples, where the input DNA concentration can be as low as 100 ng. The method developed can be accomplished in 3 days, including the initial overnight *MspI* enzyme digestion. Although the protocol has been optimized in myeloma samples, it is broadly applicable to any clinical sample, which is restricted by very low input DNA concentrations.

Key words RRBS, DNA methylation, Bisulfite conversion, Size selection, Library preparation, Next generation sequencing, Multiple myeloma

1 Introduction

Epigenetic modifications, including DNA methylation and hydroxymethylation, histone covalent modifications, and noncoding RNA mechanisms, have gained a significant amount of attention for the prevention and treatment of different genetic disorders, with cancer at the forefront [1–4]. In particular, abnormalities in genome-wide DNA methylation pattern are considered hallmarks in the majority of cancers, since it significantly contributes to the repression of tumor suppressor genes, genetic imprinting, transposable elements or X-chromosome inactivation [5–7]. A major thrust in epigenetic research is aimed at mapping the DNA methylation profile using genome-scale methods. Over the last decade, several groups have reported advanced methodologies for comprehensive methylation sequencing at the DNA level [8, 9]. Reduced

The original version of this chapter was revised. The correction to this chapter is available at https://doi.org/10.1007/978-1-4939-7865-6_17

Christoph Heuck and Niels Weinhold (eds.), *Multiple Myeloma: Methods and Protocols*, Methods in Molecular Biology, vol. 1792, https://doi.org/10.1007/978-1-4939-7865-6_13, © Springer Science+Business Media, LLC, part of Springer Nature 2018

Representation Bisulfite Sequencing (RRBS) is one of the most practiced methodologies in this context [10]. Although the maximum coverage of CpG sites does not exceed 10% of the entire human genome, RRBS is still gaining popularity for its advantage of using significantly low input DNA and cutting down the cost of high throughput sequencing [11, 12]. However, both the original and follow up modified RRBS protocols are cumbersome and require at least four working days for library preparation. This time frame makes it difficult to use for large numbers of clinical samples. Here, we have substantially modified the RRBS protocol, which can be accomplished in 3 days including the overnight digestion with *MspI*. Moreover, we have optimized a bead-based size selection method, compared to the gel-based size selection method, which facilitates DNA methylation profiling in a wide range of genomic regions with a higher throughput (Fig. 1).

Multiple Myeloma (MM) is an incurable neoplasm characterized by clonal expansion of plasma cells in the bone marrow. Onset and progression of MM from the premalignant stage monoclonal gammopathy of undetermined significance (MGUS) harbors distinct and diverse genetic anomalies such as mutations, chromosomal rearrangements, or aneusomies [13]. Simultaneously, several studies have recently reported the pivotal role of epigenetics, in particular DNA methylation, in the initiation and progression of MM [14, 15]. Despite recognizing the significant role of DNA methylation in MM, high throughput sequencing methods remain mostly restricted to gene promoters [14, 16]. The importance of DNA methylation at the intragenic regions and gene bodies has been recognized in MM [17]; however, the mechanism remains elusive due to absence of comprehensive methylome mapping. The present protocol is aimed at developing a platform for determining global DNA methylation patterns in MM cell lines and clinical isolates with an input DNA amount as low as 100 ng. Although the method has been optimized using MM samples, it could be implemented in any clinical sample. The protocol presented here allows for preparation of RRBS libraries for next generation sequencing, but not data analysis which may vary depending on the experimental design.

2 Materials

2.1 Reagents (see Note 1)

1. Bisulfite conversion kit (Zymo Research).
2. DNA cleanup and concentrator kit (Zymo Research).
3. End repair and A-tailing, adapter ligation (KAPA HyperPlus Library Preparation Kit).
4. EpiMark® Hot Start Taq DNA Polymerase (New England Biolabs Inc.).

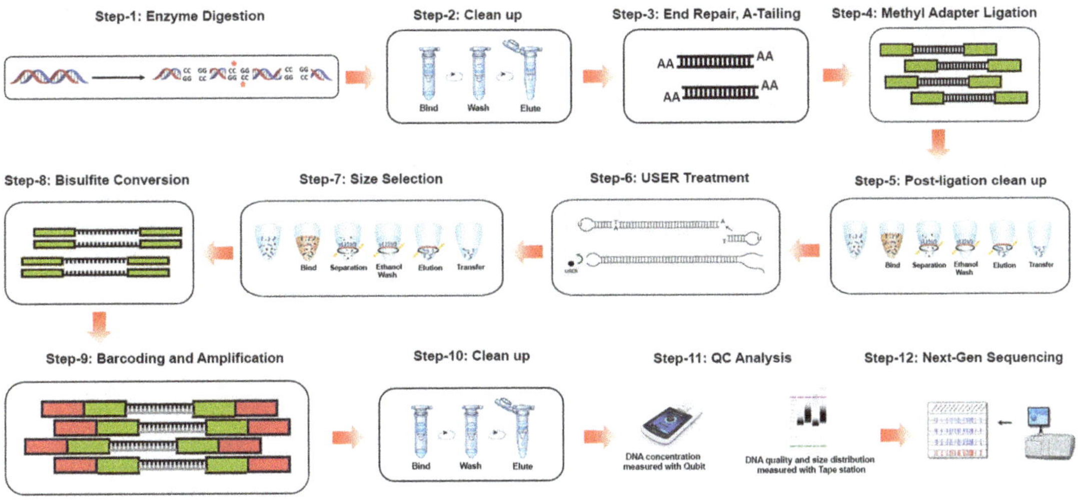

Fig. 1 Schematic illustrating the key steps involved in reduced representation bisulfite sequencing in myeloma cells

5. Ethanol (Sigma-Aldrich).
6. EZ DNA methylation kit (Zymo Research).
7. Genomic DNA sample (100–500 ng).
8. MspI (New England Biolabs Inc.).
9. NEBNext® Multiplex Oligos for Illumina® (Index Primers Sets) (New England Biolabs Inc., cat. Nos. E7335S, E7500S, E7710S, and E7730S).
10. Ultrapure water (Thermo Fisher Scientific).

2.2 Equipment (see Note 1)

1. Magnetic rack, 0.2 mL (Diagenode).
2. Magnetic separation beads (Beckman-Coulter).
3. Manual pipettes (Thermo Finnpipettes F1).
4. Microcentrifuge (Thermo Fisher Scientific).
5. Microcentrifuge tubes (USA Scientific).
6. Pipette tips (USA Scientific).
7. Qubit fluorometer (Thermo Fisher Scientific).
8. TapeStation (Agilent Technologies).
9. Thermal cycler (Thermo Fisher Scientific, ProFlex™ 96-well PCR System).
10. Thermomixer (Eppendorf).
11. Thin-walled PCR tubes, 0.2 mL (USA Scientific).
12. Vortex mixer (Thermo Fisher Scientific).

3 Methods

3.1 Digestion of Genomic DNA with MspI (▲Timing 16 h)

1. Prepare the reaction mixture for enzyme digestion as described below in a 96-well plate:

Component	Volume
Buffer (NEB 2.1)	10 μL
MspI (20 units/μL)	2 μL
Genomic DNA	X μL (100 ng)
Adjust water to	100 μL

2. Mix the reaction by brief vortexing or gentle repeated pipetting.
3. Incubate the reaction mixture in a thermocycler at 37 °C overnight (~16 h) with the heated lid set to 47°C.

3.2 Cleanup of the Digested DNA (▲Timing 10 min)

1. Thoroughly mix 100 μL of the enzyme-digested DNA to 500 μL of DNA binding buffer (1:5 ratio; Zymo), transfer to the DNA cleanup and concentrator spin-column, and centrifuge for 30 s at high speed (≥10,000 × *g*). Discard the flow-through.
2. Add 200 μL of DNA wash buffer (with added 96–100% ethanol) to the column and centrifuge for 30 s at high speed. Discard the flow-through. Repeat the step.
3. Add 55 μL of DNA elution buffer to the spin column, incubate at room temperature for 2 min, and centrifuge at high speed (*see* **Note 2**).
4. Determine the concentration of DNA from each sample using 2 μL of eluate using the Qubit fluorometer "broad-range" DNA standard solutions, per manufacturer's protocol.

3.3 End Repair and A-Tailing (▲Timing 35 min)

1. Prepare the End-repair and A-tailing reaction volume as described below.

Component	Volume (μL)
MspI-digested DNA	50
KAPA End-repair and A-tailing buffer	7
KAPA End-repair and A-tailing enzyme mix	3
Total reaction volume	**60**

2. Mix the reaction by gentle vortexing, followed by a quick spin. Incubate the sample on ice, until the thermocycler is ready for the run.

3. Incubate the samples in a thermocycler, programmed as described below (*see* **Note 3**).

Step	Temperature (°C)	Time
End-repair and A-tailing	65	30 min
Hold	4	∞

Proceed immediately to methyl adapter ligation.

3.4 Methyl Adapter Ligation (▲Timing 50 min)

1. Ligation of the methylated adapters (as supplied in NEB kits) to the end-repaired and A-tailed genomic DNAs is performed by setting up the reaction mixture, as follows.

Component	Volume (μL)
End-repair and A-tailing product	60
Undiluted methylated adapter (NEB)	4
Ultrapure water	6
Adapter ligation buffer (KAPA)	30
DNA ligase (KAPA)	10
Total reaction volume	**110**

2. Mix the reaction by gentle vortexing, followed by a quick spin. Incubate the sample on ice, until the thermocycler is ready for the run.
3. Incubate the samples in a thermocycler programmed as described below (*see* **Note 3**).

Step	Temperature (°C)	Time
Adapter ligation	20	45 min
Hold	4	∞

3.5 Postligation Cleanup (▲Timing 30 min)

1. Add 0.8× magnetic beads to the adapter-ligated libraries as below:

Component	Volume (μL)
Adapter-ligated reaction product	110
Agencourt AMPure XP reagent	88
Total reaction volume	**198**

2. Thoroughly mix the samples with gentle vortexing or by pipetting up and down multiple times.
3. Incubate the tubes at room temperature for 15 min to allow adequate binding of library molecules to the beads.
4. Transfer the tubes to a magnetic rack and incubate the tubes for ~5 min.
5. Open the tube and carefully remove the supernatant. Perform this in two steps, first by removing 190 μL then removing the last 10 μL to prevent removal of beads.
6. Keeping the tube in the magnetic rack, add 200 μL of freshly prepared 80% ethanol.
7. Incubate the tubes in rack for 30 s.
8. Carefully remove the ethanol without disturbing the beads.
9. Repeat the ethanol wash step.
10. Carefully remove and discard the ethanol from the tubes and air-dry the beads for 5 min. Over drying may result in loss of DNA and should be avoided (*see* **Note 6**).
11. Remove the tubes from the magnetic rack and add 55 μL of DNA elution buffer and mix thoroughly with the beads by pipetting up and down multiple times.
12. Incubate at room temperature for 2 min to elute the DNA from the beads.
13. Transfer the tubes to the magnetic rack to capture the beads. Incubate the tubes in rack for 5 min.
14. Carefully transfer ~50 μL of the supernatant to a new tube. Two transfers of 40 μL and 10 μL will prevent transfer of beads.

Safe Stopping Point: The purified and post-ligated library molecules can be stored at − 20 °C for 1–2 weeks.

3.6 USER Enzyme Treatment (▲ Timing 20 min)

1. Add 1.5 μL of Uracil-Specific Excision Reagent (USER) to the DNA samples from Subheading 3.5, **step 13** and mix thoroughly by pipetting multiple times up and down (*see* **Note 4**).
2. Incubate the samples in a thermocycler programmed as described below (*see* **Note 3**).

Step	Temperature (°C)	Time
USER reaction	15	15 min
Hold	4	∞

3.7 Size Selection (▲ Timing 40 min)

A "dual" size selection method is followed to obtain libraries with fragments sized between <250 bp and 250–450 bp.

1. Incubate the DNA Sample with 0.6× Beads as below (*see* **Note 6**):

Component	Volume (μL)
DNA to be size selected	50
Agencourt AMPure XP reagent	30
Total reaction volume	**80**

2. Thoroughly mix the samples with gentle vortexing or by pipetting up and down multiple times.
3. Incubate the tubes at room temperature for 15 min to allow binding of library molecules >450 bp to the beads.
4. Transfer the tubes to a magnetic rack to capture the beads. Incubate the tubes in the rack for 5 min.
5. Carefully transfer ~75 μL of the supernatant containing library molecules smaller than 450 bp to a new tube. Discard the tubes with magnetic beads (*see* **Note 5**). Continue to the second step of the size selection with the supernatant.
6. The second size selection step involved incubation with 0.1× magnetic beads with the DNA samples as below (*see* **Note 6**):

Component	Volume (μL)
Supernatant from the first size-cut	75
Agencourt AMPure XP reagent	10
Total reaction volume	**85**

7. Thoroughly mix the samples with gentle vortexing or by pipetting up and down multiple times.
8. Incubate the tubes at room temperature for 15 min to allow binding of library molecules >250 bp to the beads.
9. Transfer the tubes to the magnetic rack to capture the beads. Incubate the tubes in the rack for 5 min.
10. Carefully transfer ~75 μL of the supernatant containing library molecules smaller than 250 bp, to a new tube and store in ice for further clean up. Keep the tubes with magnetic beads. It is crucial to monitor that no beads are transferred along with the supernatant.
11. Keeping the tube in the magnetic rack, add 200 μL of freshly prepared 80% ethanol.
12. Incubate the tubes in rack for 5 min.
13. Carefully remove the ethanol without disturbing the beads.
14. Repeat the ethanol wash step.

15. Carefully remove and discard the ethanol from the tubes and air-dry the beads for 5 min. Over drying may results in loss of DNA and should be avoided (*see* **Note 7**).
16. Remove the tubes from the magnetic racks and add 40 μL of DNA-elution buffer and mix thoroughly by pipetting up and down multiple times.
17. Incubate at room temperature for 2 min to elute the library molecules from the beads.
18. Transfer the tubes to the magnetic rack to capture the beads. Incubate the tubes in the rack for 5 min.
19. Carefully transfer ~40 μL of the supernatant containing library molecules sized between 250 and 450 bp to a new tube and store in ice.
20. Thoroughly mix 375 μL (5 volumes) of DNA binding buffer to the supernatant (75 μL) of 10, and pass through the DNA clean up column, and centrifuge for 30 s at high speed (≥10,000 × *g*).
21. Add 200 μL of DNA wash buffer to the column and centrifuge for 30 s at high speed. Repeat the step.
22. Add 40 μL of DNA elution buffer to the spin column, incubate at room temperature for 2 min, and centrifuge at high speed (*see* **Note 2**). The eluate contains library molecules sized lower than 250 bp.

Safe Stopping Point: The purified and size-selected library molecules can be stored at −20 °C for 1–2 weeks.

3.8 Bisulfite Conversion (▲ Timing 16 h)

1. Add 5 μL of M-dilution buffer (EZ DNA methylation kit) and 5 μL of water to each of the DNA fractions (sized lower than 250 bp and between 250 and 450 bp respectively), and incubate at 37 °C for 15 min.
2. Meanwhile, prepare the bisulfite conversion (CT) reagent by mixing 210 μL of Mdilution buffer and 750 μL of ultrapure water to the content of CT-reagents per vial (*see* **Note 7**).
3. Add 100 μL of the CT conversion reagent to each sample and incubate in a thermocycler as programmed below.

Step	Temperature (°C)	Time	
Denaturation	95	30 s	55 cycles
Bisulfite conversion	50	15 min	
Hold	4	>10 min	

4. Thoroughly mix 400 μL of M-binding buffer to the bisulfite converted DNA from 3.8.3, and pass through a spin column at high speed for 30 s. Discard the flow-through.

5. Add 200 μL of M-wash buffer and centrifuge at high speed for 30 s. Discard the flow-through.
6. Add 200 μL of M-desulfonation buffer to the column and incubate for 15–20 min at room temperature.
7. Centrifuge at high speed for 30 s. Discard the flow-through.
8. Add 200 μL of M-wash buffer, centrifuge at high speed for 1 min. Discard the flow through. Repeat the washing step.
9. Elute the DNA with 40 μL of water. Incubate for 1 min and centrifuge at high speed (*see* **Note 2**).

3.9 Barcoding and Amplification of Libraries (▲ Timing 40 min)

1. This step enriches the library molecules that are ligated to the methylated adapters at both the ends.
2. The enrichment PCR is performed from both fractions (less than 250 bp and between 250 and 450 bp). Each fraction is divided into two PCR reactions. Each fraction derived from one sample should have the same index primer, but different samples should have different indexes to allow for multiplexing on the sequencer. The reaction set up is described below for each sample (×2).

Component	Volume (μL)
Adapter-ligated, bisulfite-converted DNA	20
NEBNext universal PCR primer	2.5
NEBNext index (X) primer	2.5
5× EpiMark Hotstart Taq reaction buffer	10
10 mM dNTPs (NEB)	1
Epimark Hotstart Taq (2 units/μL)	0.25
Ultrapure water	13.75
Total reaction volume	**50**

3. The PCR amplification is performed in a thermocycler, as programmed below.

Step	Temperature (°C)	Time	Cycles
Denaturation	95	30 s	1
Cycling	90	15 s	15
	61	30 s	
	68	30 s	
Hold	4	∞	1

3.10 Cleanup of the Amplified Libraries (▲ Timing 10 min)

1. Thoroughly mix 50 μL of the PCR product with 250 μL of DNA binding buffer (1:5 ratio), transfer to a spin-column, and centrifuge for 30 s at high speed (≥10,000 × *g*). Discard the flow-through.
2. Add 200 μL of DNA wash buffer to the column and centrifuge for 30 s at high speed. Discard the flow-through. Repeat the step.
3. Add 20 μL of DNA elution buffer (96–100% ethanol supplemented) to the spin column, incubate at room temperature for 2 min, and centrifuge at high speed (*see* **Note 2**).

3.11 QC Analysis of the Libraries (▲ Timing 15 min)

1. Determine the concentration of the final library molecules from both the lower (<250 bp) and upper fractions (250–450 bp) using Qubit fluorometer with 2 μL of each sample against the high-sensitivity DNA standard solutions.
2. Simultaneously, determine the purity and size distribution of the library fractions using the Tapestation with 2 μL of each sample, mixed in 2 μL of high sensitivity buffer solutions, per manufacturer's protocol. The difference and distribution of DNA fragment size should be compared to the pattern, as represented with the example of two myeloma cell lines (H929 and KMS12BM) in Fig. 2.
3. Determine the average size of each fraction using the Tapestation.
4. The average size (in bp) from Tape station and the concentration of libraries (ng), as obtained from the Qubit will be used to measure the molarity of each fragment.
5. Prepare 10 μL of 2 nM solution of each lower (library size less than 250 bp) and upper (between 250 and 450 bp) fraction by diluting with ultrapure water.

Calculation of Molarity
Nanomolar concentration of DNA = [(concentration of DNA/1000)/(Average size of library fraction*660)]*10^9.
Concentration of DNA: As obtained from Qubit.
Average size of library fraction: As obtained from TapeStation data.
660: Weight of standard double standard DNA base pair.

6. Pool and mix 10 μL of 2 nM solution of each lower and upper fraction to prepare the final RRBS library. Libraries should be sequenced to at least 20 million reads using single end

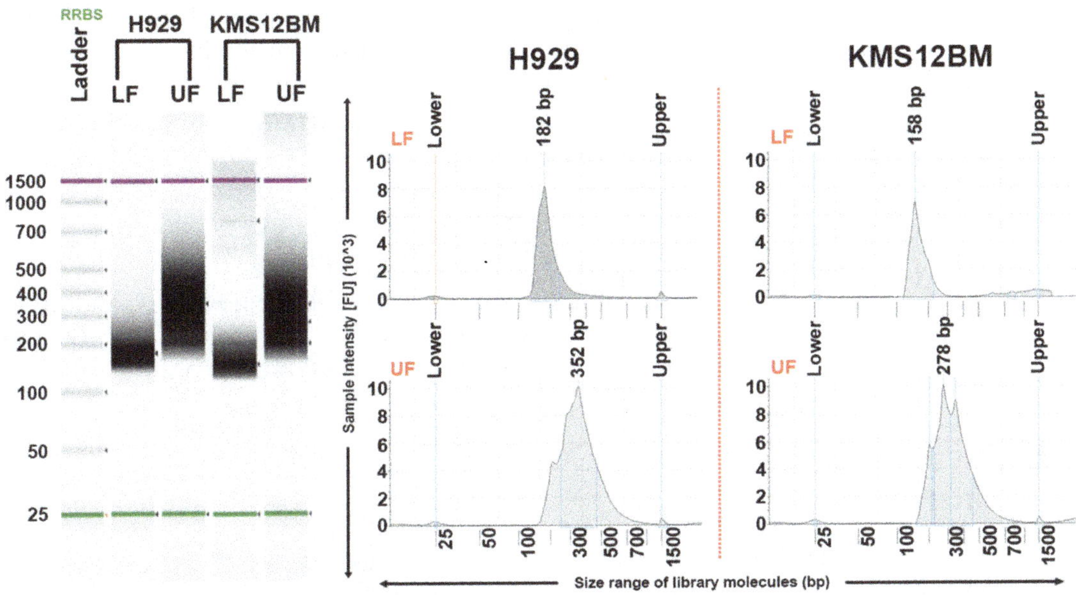

Fig. 2 Size distribution of lower (<250 bp) and upper fraction (250–450 bp) of the final library molecules, as visualized with TapeStation

50–75 bp reads. Due to low complexity of RRBS libraries, 30% PhiX control (or other high complexity library) should be spiked in to prevent sequencing run failure.

7. Acquisition and analysis of RRBS data can be performed by following the guidelines, as available in the standard literature [18–21]

4 Notes

1. The present protocol has been optimized with the reagents and equipment from the manufacturers, as mentioned the "Materials and Method" section. Similar products from other manufacturers might work as well, but may be subjected to optimization by the respective users.
2. In all the elution steps, passing the elution buffer/ water through the column for second time would give higher yield of DNA.
3. It should be noted that the temperature of the lid should be ~85 °C, instead of 105 °C. This prevents overheating and degradation of the samples.
4. USER treatment creates a cleavage at the uracil (U) residue in the hairpin structure of the methylated adapter. This causes the DNA ends to form a fork structure that facilitates the PCR amplification during library enrichment.

5. It's crucial to monitor that no beads are transferred along with the supernatants. Performing the transfer in two steps will minimize bead transfer.
6. The first size cut uses 0.6× of Agencourt AMPure XP reagent to the target DNA volume, i.e., 30 μL of reagent to 50 μL of DNA solution. The second cut uses a 0.2× of the reagent of initial volume of DNA solution (50 μL) to the supernatant (75 μL) from the first cut, i.e., 10 μL.
7. Use 0.2–10 μL microtips for carefully removing ethanol from the beads. The suction/cohesion action of the microtips should remove the alcohol droplets from the beads.

References

1. Esteller M (2008) Epigenetics in cancer. N Engl J Med 358(11):1148–1159. https://doi.org/10.1056/NEJMra072067
2. Egger G, Liang G, Aparicio A, Jones PA (2004) Epigenetics in human disease and prospects for epigenetic therapy. Nature 429(6990):457–463
3. Laird PW, Jaenisch R (1996) The role of DNA methylation in cancer genetic and epigenetics. Annu Rev Genet 30:441–464. https://doi.org/10.1146/annurev.genet.30.1.441
4. Choudhury SR, Cui Y, Lubecka K, Stefanska B, Irudayaraj J (2016) CRISPR-dCas9 mediated TET1 targeting for selective DNA demethylation at BRCA1 promoter. Oncotarget 7(29):46545–46556. https://doi.org/10.18632/oncotarget.10234
5. Lister R, Pelizzola M, Dowen RH, Hawkins RD, Hon G, Tonti-Filippini J, Nery JR, Lee L, Ye Z, Ngo Q-M, Edsall L, Antosiewicz-Bourget J, Stewart R, Ruotti V, Millar AH, Thomson JA, Ren B, Ecker JR (2009) Human DNA methylomes at base resolution show widespread epigenomic differences. Nature 462(7271):315–322. http://www.nature.com/nature/journal/v462/n7271/suppinfo/nature08514_S1.html
6. Bird A (2002) DNA methylation patterns and epigenetic memory. Genes Dev 16(1):6–21. https://doi.org/10.1101/gad.947102
7. Li E, Beard C, Jaenisch R (1993) Role for DNA methylation in genomic imprinting. Nature 366(6453):362–365. https://doi.org/10.1038/366362a0
8. Weber M, Davies JJ, Wittig D, Oakeley EJ, Haase M, Lam WL, Schubeler D (2005) Chromosome-wide and promoter-specific analyses identify sites of differential DNA methylation in normal and transformed human cells. Nat Genet 37(8):853–862. http://www.nature.com/ng/journal/v37/n8/suppinfo/ng1598_S1.html
9. Meissner A, Mikkelsen TS, Gu H, Wernig M, Hanna J, Sivachenko A, Zhang X, Bernstein BE, Nusbaum C, Jaffe DB, Gnirke A, Jaenisch R, Lander ES (2008) Genome-scale DNA methylation maps of pluripotent and differentiated cells. Nature 454(7205):766–770. http://www.nature.com/nature/journal/v454/n7205/suppinfo/nature07107_S1.html
10. Meissner A, Gnirke A, Bell GW, Ramsahoye B, Lander ES, Jaenisch R (2005) Reduced representation bisulfite sequencing for comparative high-resolution DNA methylation analysis. Nucleic Acids Res 33(18):5868–5877. https://doi.org/10.1093/nar/gki901
11. Gu H, Bock C, Mikkelsen TS, Jager N, Smith ZD, Tomazou E, Gnirke A, Lander ES, Meissner A (2010) Genome-scale DNA methylation mapping of clinical samples at single-nucleotide resolution. Nat Methods 7(2):133–136. https://doi.org/10.1038/nmeth.1414
12. Guo H, Zhu P, Yan L, Li R, Hu B, Lian Y, Yan J, Ren X, Lin S, Li J, Jin X, Shi X, Liu P, Wang X, Wang W, Wei Y, Li X, Guo F, Wu X, Fan X, Yong J, Wen L, Xie SX, Tang F, Qiao J (2014) The DNA methylation landscape of human early embryos. Nature 511(7511):606–610. https://doi.org/10.1038/nature13544. http://www.nature.com/nature/journal/v511/n7511/abs/nature13544.html#supplementary-information
13. Morgan GJ, Walker BA, Davies FE (2012) The genetic architecture of multiple myeloma. Nat Rev Cancer 12(5):335–348. https://doi.org/10.1038/nrc3257
14. Walker BA, Wardell CP, Chiecchio L, Smith EM, Boyd KD, Neri A, Davies FE, Ross FM, Morgan GJ (2011) Aberrant global methyla-

tion patterns affect the molecular pathogenesis and prognosis of multiple myeloma. Blood 117(2):553–562. https://doi.org/10.1182/blood-2010-04-279539

15. Kaiser MF, Johnson DC, Wu P, Walker BA, Brioli A, Mirabella F, Wardell CP, Melchor L, Davies FE, Morgan GJ (2013) Global methylation analysis identifies prognostically important epigenetically inactivated tumor suppressor genes in multiple myeloma. Blood 122(2):219–226. https://doi.org/10.1182/blood-2013-03-487884
16. Salhia B, Baker A, Ahmann G, Auclair D, Fonsa R, Carpten J (2010) DNA methylation analysis determines the high frequency of genic hypomethylation and low frequency of hypermethylation events in plasma cell tumors. Cancer Res 70(17):6934–6944. https://doi.org/10.1158/0008-5472.can-10-0282
17. Bollati V, Fabris S, Pegoraro V, Ronchetti D, Mosca L, Deliliers GL, Motta V, Bertazzi PA, Baccarelli A, Neri A (2009) Differential repetitive DNA methylation in multiple myeloma molecular subgroups. Carcinogenesis 30(8):1330–1335. https://doi.org/10.1093/carcin/bgp149
18. Wang T, Liu Q, Li X, Wang X, Li J, Zhu X, Sun ZS, Wu J (2013) RRBS-analyser: a comprehensive web server for reduced representation bisulfite sequencing data analysis. Hum Mutat 34(12):1606–1610. https://doi.org/10.1002/humu.22444
19. Xi Y, Bock C, Muller F, Sun D, Meissner A, Li W (2012) RRBSMAP: a fast, accurate and user-friendly alignment tool for reduced representation bisulfite sequencing. Bioinformatics 28(3):430–432. https://doi.org/10.1093/bioinformatics/btr668
20. Krueger F, Andrews SR (2011) Bismark: a flexible aligner and methylation caller for bisulfite-Seq applications. Bioinformatics 27(11):1571–1572. https://doi.org/10.1093/bioinformatics/btr167
21. Li H, Handsaker B, Wysoker A, Fennell T, Ruan J, Homer N, Marth G, Abecasis G, Durbin R (2009) The sequence alignment/map format and SAMtools. Bioinformatics 25(16):2078–2079. https://doi.org/10.1093/bioinformatics/btp352

Chapter 14

Microfluidic Production and Application of Lipid Nanoparticles for Nucleic Acid Transfection

Anitha Thomas, Shyam M. Garg, Rebecca A. G. De Souza, Eric Ouellet, Grace Tharmarajah, Dave Reichert, Mina Ordobadi, Shell Ip, and Euan C. Ramsay

Abstract

Lipid nanoparticles (LNPs) are established in the biopharmaceutical industry for efficient encapsulation and cytosolic delivery of nucleic acids for potential therapeutics, with several formulations in clinical trials. The advantages of LNPs can also be applied in basic research and discovery with a microfluidic method of preparation now commercially available that allows preparations to be scaled down to quantities appropriate for cell culture. These preparations conserve expensive nucleic acids while maintaining the particle characteristics that have made LNPs successful in later stages of genetic medicine development. Additionally, this method and the resulting LNPs are seamlessly scalable to quantities appropriate for in vivo models and development of nucleic acid therapeutics.

The present work describes the methodology for preparing LNPs loaded with siRNA, mRNA or plasmids using a commercially available microfluidic instrument and an accompanying transfection kit. Guidelines for application to cultured cells in a well-plate format are also provided.

Key words Transfection, Lipid nanoparticle, RNAi, siRNA, mRNA, Plasmid, Encapsulation

1 Introduction

Lipid nanoparticles (LNPs) are used extensively by the biopharmaceutical industry to deliver genetic medicines currently in preclinical and clinical development. They offer high nucleic acid encapsulation efficiency and potent transfection with low cytotoxicity and immunogenicity [1]. Microfluidic systems are the best available method for producing LNPs, as microfluidics allows for scalable, high-throughput production of nucleic acid-containing LNPs. Nucleic acid-containing LNPs self-assemble during microfluidic mixing when an aqueous stream containing the nucleic acid is rapidly mixed with an ethanol stream containing structural lipids, ionizable cationic lipids, polyethylene glycol-conjugated (PEGylated) lipids, and cholesterol. Targeting moieties can also be

Christoph Heuck and Niels Weinhold (eds.), *Multiple Myeloma: Methods and Protocols*, Methods in Molecular Biology, vol. 1792, https://doi.org/10.1007/978-1-4939-7865-6_14, © Springer Science+Business Media, LLC, part of Springer Nature 2018

incorporated onto the LNP surface to facilitate the delivery of the nucleic acid payload to the appropriate cells. Commercial systems such as the NanoAssemblr™ platform have recently become available to enable users to consistently produce nucleic acid LNPs at scales appropriate for basic research through to clinical development.

In contrast with lipoplexes, which are cationic liposomes complexed with nucleic acids, LNPs are smaller and nontoxic. The incorporation of PEGylated lipids into LNPs allows them to reach sizes well below 100 nm in diameter [2]: much smaller than the 1000 nm size limit for lipoplexes. In addition to decreasing LNP size, surface PEGylation resists the adsorption of serum proteins, both of which improve LNP penetration into tumor tissues to deliver therapeutics. Additionally, lipoplexes are made from cationic lipids, which both bind the anionic nucleic acids and destabilize cell membranes to allow lipoplexes to be absorbed. These cationic lipids are highly cytotoxic and immunogenic [3], whereas the ionizable cationic lipids used to produce LNPs are neutral at physiological pH and LNPs are absorbed by receptor-mediated endocytosis, which greatly improves cell viability and allows in vivo administration (Fig. 1). Furthermore, nucleic acids in LNPs are completely encapsulated within the core of the particle, which protects them from degradation by extracellular nucleases.

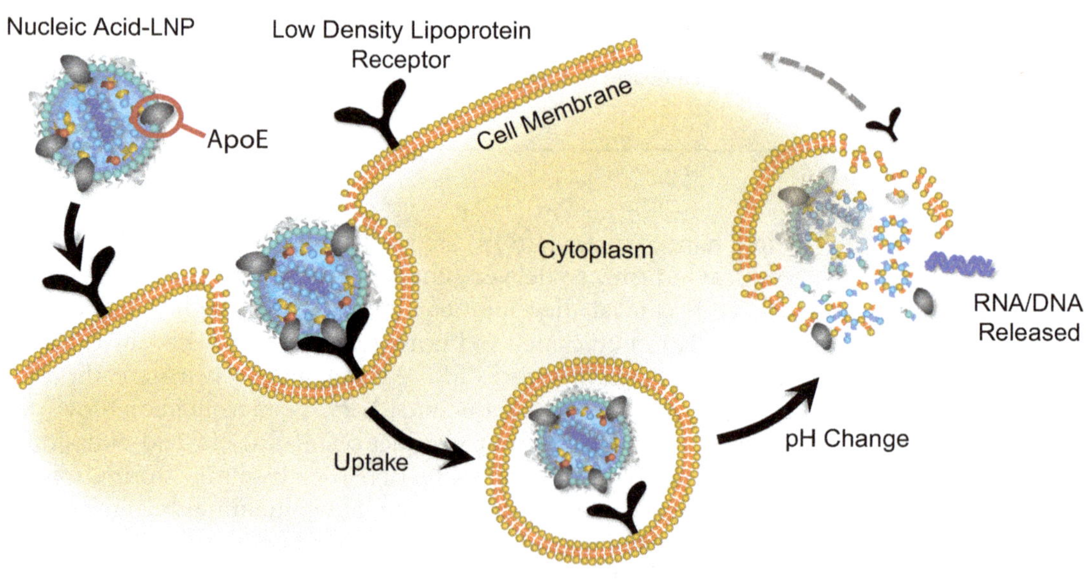

Fig. 1 Lipid nanoparticles resemble low density lipoproteins (LDL) and are taken up by receptor-mediated endocytosis governed by the LDL receptor present on many cell types and Apolipoprotein-E. In the endosome, acidic conditions cause the pH-sensitive ionizable lipids to become cationic where they disrupt the endosome and release their nucleic acid payload

1.1 LNPs Established in Genetic Medicine

LNPs have proven their worth in delivering therapeutic nucleic acids for the treatment of blood diseases, including cancer. LNPs produced by the NanoAssemblr microfluidic mixing device from Precision NanoSystems have already been used to deliver tumor-suppressive microRNAs, including *let-7* [4] and *mir-124* [5], to treat cancer in animal models. Researchers discovered that delivering *let-7* inhibited the proliferation of *MYC*-driven hepatoblastoma and that *mir-124* was a potent inhibitor of the STAT3 pathway, which plays a key role in tumor-mediated immune suppression. LNPs could also potentially be used to deliver mRNA coding for the chimeric antigen receptors (CARs) used in CAR T-cell therapy treatments for myeloma, which avoids potential issues from using viral vectors such as laborious preparation, and potential immunogenicity and safety concerns.

Nevertheless, delivering RNA to blood cancer cells remains difficult, due to both the systemic distribution of these cells and the inherent difficulty of transfecting them while avoiding an immune response. Coating the surface of LNPs with monoclonal antibodies (mAbs) against leukocyte cell surface receptors is one method that has been successfully used to achieve targeted RNA delivery to specific leukocyte subsets [6]. Systemic administration of LNPs modified with mAbs against the CD38 receptor found on most mantle cell lymphomas (MCLs) were successfully used to deliver siRNA to the bone marrow to treat human MCL in a mouse xenograft model [7]. This illustrates the importance of appropriate targeting in effectively utilizing LNPs for the clinical treatment of blood cancers.

1.2 Application of Lipid Nanoparticles in Basic Research and Discovery

LNPs also have significant application in basic research and discovery. Specifically, LNPs have been used to elucidate the effects of microRNA expression in primary motor neurons through high-content screening (HCS) [8]. HCS allows for the phenotypic changes in cells treated with nucleic acids delivered by LNPs to be precisely quantified while reducing experimental variability by maintaining constant culture conditions. HCS platforms allow gene regulation to be investigated in a high-throughput manner, to rapidly validate gene function, discover new therapeutic targets, or optimize oligonucleotide sequences.

These examples illustrate how LNPs produced by microfluidics have been utilized in basic research and applied in the development of genetic medicines for B-cell cancers. This protocol outlines the preparation of nucleic acid LNPs using a commercially available microfluidic instrument and an associated transfection kit (Fig. 2). This protocol also covers the treatment of plated cells with the resulting LNP suspensions. These nucleic acid LNPs have been used successfully in animal models and have promising results in clinical trials, and therefore show clear potential for use as a delivery vehicle for genetic medicines.

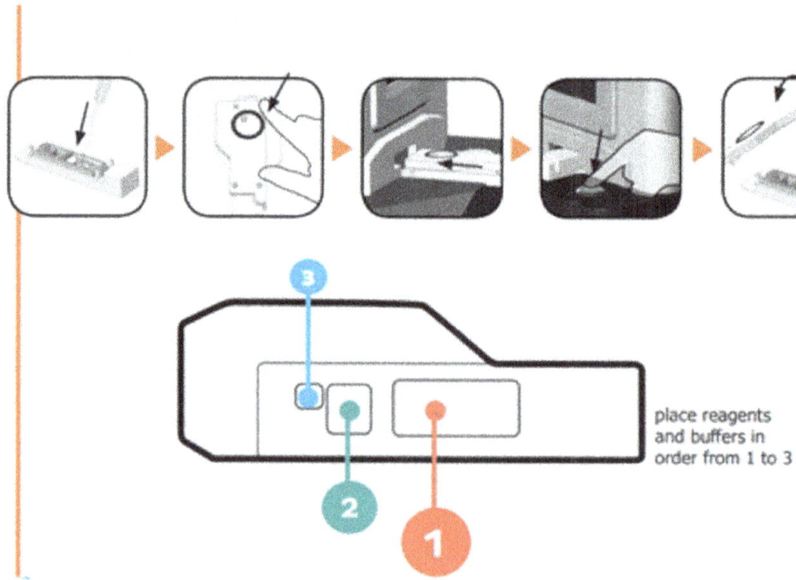

Fig. 2 Illustrations outlining the process for preparing nucleic acid–LNPs using Spark Transfection Kits. Well 1 is filled with 48 μL of Spark Formulation Buffer 2 prior to the formulation, while well 2 is filled with 36 μL of the nucleic acid in Formulation Buffer 1 and well 1 is filled with 12 μL of the Spark Nanoparticle Mix. The filled cartridge is capped and placed in the Spark to manufacture the nanoparticles. The final nanoparticle product is in well 1 once the encapsulation is complete

2 Materials

1. Nucleic acid to be encapsulated
   (a) 2 nmol siRNA, lyophilized (Integrated DNA Technologies, USA)
   OR
   (b) 20 μg mRNA, at least 1 mg/mL in buffer (TriLink BioTechnologies, USA),
   OR
   (c) 15 μg plasmid DNA, at least 1 mg/mL (concentrated, of high purity, and endotoxin free).
2. Recombinant Human Apolipoprotein-E4 (ApoE4) (Peprotech, USA).
3. Nuclease-free filter tips (10, 20, 200, and 1000 μL).
4. Nuclease-free microcentrifuge tubes (1.5 mL).
5. Micropipettes, 10, 20, 200, and 1000 μL (general supplier).
6. RNAseZAP™ for RNA encapsulation (Sigma-Aldrich, USA).
7. NanoAssemblr™ Spark™ (Precision NanoSystems Inc., Canada).
8. Spark Transfection kit.

   (a) Spark microfluidic cartridge.
   (b) Corresponding Spark Nanoparticle Mix.
   (c) Corresponding Spark Formulation Buffer 1.
   (d) Corresponding Spark Formulation Buffer 2.
9. Synergy H1 Multi-Mode Microplate Reader (Biotek, USA).
10. NanoDrop™ 2000c UV-Vis spectrometer (ThermoFisher Scientific, USA).
11. Cells of interest, plated according to user protocols and for downstream analysis of interest.
12. Fluorescence microscope or a flow cytometer for cell treatment analysis.

3 Methods

3.1 Nucleic Acid Sample Preparation

1. Thaw and spin down the nucleic acid sample and Buffers. Mix thawed Formulation Buffers thoroughly by vortexing or pipetting up and down multiple times (*see* **Notes 1–3**). Starting quantities and typical concentrations for siRNA, mRNA and plasmid DNA are indicated in Table 1.
   (a) If working with 2 nmol lyophilized siRNA, skip to 3.1.2. OR
   (b) If working with previously reconstituted siRNA, or mRNA or plasmid, mix thawed samples and skip to 3.1.3.
2. Reconstitute siRNA by pipetting Spark Formulation Buffer 1 into the siRNA sample tube following Table 2 (*see* **Note 3**).
3. If diluting nucleic acid samples, pipette the volume of the nucleic acid sample prescribed in Table 2 into a nuclease-free microcentrifuge tube and add the corresponding quantity of Spark Formulation Buffer 1 into the same tube (*see* **Note 4**).
4. Confirm final concentration via NanoDrop 2000 c UV-Vis spectrophotometer or a traditional spectrophotometer and adjust the concentration to match the last line of Table 2 if needed.

Table 1
Starting Quantities for different nucleic acid payloads

	siRNA	mRNA	Plasmid
Nominal quantity	2 nmol siRNA[a]	20 µg	15 µg
Recommended starting concentration	Lyophilized 20 mg/mL in nuclease-free water	1 mg/mL (from supplier, in Tris–HCl or citrate buffer)	1 mg/mL (from midi prep in TE buffer—10 mM Tris +1 mM disodium EDTA)

[a]If lyophilized siRNA is >2 nmol, reconstitute to 20 mg/mL in nuclease-free water. *See* **Note 3**

Table 2
Preparation for NanoAssemblr Spark formulation

	siRNA		mRNA	Plasmid DNA
Starting concentration	Lyophilized	20 mg/mL stock	1 mg/mL	1 mg/mL
Volume of nucleic acid solution (μL)	N/A	1.8	22	13.4
Volume of corresponding FB1[a] (μL)	36	37.2	17.6	23
Total volume (μL)	36	39	39.6	36.4
Target concentration[b] (mg/mL, ± 0.01 mg/mL)	0.930		0.556	0.370

[a]FB1 = Spark Formulation Buffer 1
[b]Target concentration can vary depending on the kit. Please make sure to follow kit-specific guidelines

Table 3
Estimates of Spark Kits final nucleic acid concentrations

	siRNA	mRNA	Plasmid DNA
Nominal final concentration (μg/mL)[a]	130	75	65

[a]Final LNP concentrations refer to the mass of nucleic acids per unit volume of LNP suspension and is estimated by the kit manufacturer based on multiple quantification assays. Concentrations can vary depending on the type of kit. Please make sure to follow kit-specific guidelines

3.2 Lipid Nanoparticle Formulation Using the NanoAssemblr Spark Kits

1. Place the NanoAssemblr Spark inside the biosafety cabinet and, following the instructions in the user guide, connect the instrument to the power supply and turn the instrument on.
2. Pipette 96 μL of mRNA Spark Formulation Buffer 2 into a nuclease-free microcentrifuge tube. Set this tube aside for the final dilution step after running the materials through the instrument.
3. Inside the biosafety cabinet, open the Spark Cartridge package and the accompanying Cartridge Cap. Figure 2 provides a schematic of the Spark Cartridge and the order of loading materials into the cartridge wells.
4. Pipette 48 μL of Spark Formulation Buffer 2 into the largest well of the Spark Cartridge (Well 1) (*see* **Notes 4** and **5**).
5. Pipette 36 μL of nucleic acid sample prepared in Subheading 3.1 into the middle well (Well 2) of the cartridge (*see* **Note 5**).
6. Pipette 12 μL of Nanoparticle Mix into the smallest well (Well 3) (*see* **Notes 5** and **6**).

7. Place Cartridge Cap over the base of the Cartridge and insert into the instrument, following the instructions in the Spark User Guide.
8. Press the green-lit "Start" button on the base of the instrument.
9. Once the instrument completes its process (~3 s), remove the cartridge from the instrument and lift the Cap carefully.
10. Using a pipette, remove the entire contents from Well 1 of the cartridge and add it to the microcentrifuge tube containing 96 μL of the formulation buffer 2 prepared in Subheading 3.2, **step 2**. This is the final nanoparticle product and estimated nucleic acid concentration for each payload can be found in Table 3 (*see* **Note 7**).

3.3 Nanoparticle Storage

Nanoparticles generated using the NanoAssemblr Spark have a shelf life of 14 days when stored at 4 °C. Do not vortex, heat or freeze the nanoparticles as these processes can significantly compromise particle integrity. The Spark Kit nanoparticles are labeled with a fluorescent dye for detection purposes, so keep the nanoparticles away from light.

3.4 Cell Culture for Nanoparticle Treatment

1. Plate cells as you normally would for your desired downstream assay. It is recommended that for treatment times lasting for 24–48 h, please plan your seeding densities accordingly for your desired downstream assay and for the time required for treatment, keeping in mind media changes and cell proliferation rates.
2. It is recommended to treat cells with at least three concentrations of nanoparticles to demonstrate a dose-dependent response. A titration of 0.01–1 μg/mL nucleic acid is suggested in most cases. It is also recommended to treat some wells with the relevant nucleic acid control (i.e., noncoding siRNA) as well as leaving a few wells untreated for negative controls.

3.5 Preparation of ApoE4 (*see* Note 8)

1. Thaw and spin down the lyophilized ApoE4 (50 μg).
2. Pipette 500 μL of DPBS (without Mg^{2+} and Ca^{2+}) into the tube containing lyophilized ApoE4.
3. Pipette the solution up and down (>3 times) to mix.
4. Pulse spin down the solution.
5. Relabel tube as Stock ApoE4 with the concentration 100 μg/mL (*see* **Note 9**).

3.6 Treatment of Cells in Culture

A sample experimental plan can be found in Fig. 3 and Table 4.

1. Pipette the premade nanoparticles up and down (>3 times) to mix and pulse spin down the tube. For nucleic acid concentration refer to Table 3 (*see* **Note 1**).
2. Treat the appropriate wells with the LNPs as detailed in Fig. 3 and Table 4.

Table 4
Example treatment plan for treating cells with siRNA–LNP Spark Kit nanoparticles

Well number	Well color	Treatment name	Nucleic acid–LNP dose (μg/mL)	ApoE Dose (μg/mL)	Media volume (mL)	Nanoparticle volume to add (μL)	Stock ApoE volume to add (μL)	Treatment time (h)
1A	Grey	Untreated Sample-1	0	1	1	0.0	10	48
2A	Grey	Untreated Sample-2	0	1	1	0.0	10	48
3A	Grey	Untreated Sample-3	0	1	1	0.0	10	48
4A	Blue	Treatment A Sample-1	1	0	1	7.7	0	48
5A	Blue	Treatment A Sample-2	1	0	1	7.7	0	48
6A	Blue	Treatment A Sample-3	1	0	1	7.7	0	48
1B	Green	Treatment B Sample-1	1	1	1	7.7	10	48
2B	Green	Treatment B Sample-2	1	1	1	7.7	10	48
3B	Green	Treatment B Sample-3	1	1	1	7.7	10	48
4B	Orange	Treatment C Sample-1	0.5	1	1	3.8	10	48
5B	Orange	Treatment C Sample-2	0.5	1	1	3.8	10	48
6B	Orange	Treatment C Sample-3	0.5	1	1	3.8	10	48
1C	Red	Treatment D Sample-1	0.1	1	1	0.8	10	48
2C	Red	Treatment D Sample-2	0.1	1	1	0.8	10	48
3C	Red	Treatment D Sample-3	0.1	1	1	0.8	10	48
4C	Purple	Noncoding control Sample-1	1	1	1	7.7	10	48

(continued)

Table 4 (continued)

Well number	Well color	Treatment name	Nucleic acid–LNP dose (μg/mL)	ApoE Dose (μg/mL)	Media volume (mL)	Nanoparticle volume to add (μL)	Stock ApoE volume to add (μL)	Treatment time (h)
5C	Purple	Noncoding control Sample-2	1	1	1	7.7	10	48
6C	Purple	Noncoding control Sample-3	1	1	1	7.7	10	48

Nucleic acid–LNP doses are expressed in μg nucleic acid per mL of media, and volumes of nanoparticle suspension and ApoE are calculated using the dilution formula $V_1 = C_2 \bullet V_2 \div C_1$. V1 is the volume of nucleic acid–LNP suspension required for treatment. Estimations for C_1 depend on the kit and are provided in Table 3. C_2 is the desired nucleic acid–LNP Dose and V_2 is approximately the Media Volume

3. Treat the appropriate wells with the Stock ApoE4 solution, as detailed in Fig. 3 and Table 4 (*see* **Note 10**).
4. Following treatment, gently rock the plate in a figure-eight motion to evenly distribute ApoE and LNP.
5. Process cells for desired downstream assay (e.g., fluorescent microscopy or flow cytometry) after 24–72 h using a previously validated protocol (*see* **Note 11**).

4 Notes

1. All the steps listed in methods section need to be performed in the biosafety cabinet to avoid sample contamination. Apply aseptic technique when handling the material and kit components. The particles generated through this method will be sterile and safe to use on cell cultures. Additionally, mRNA is susceptible to degradation via nucleases and thus it is crucial to work with RNAse-free labware and clean working surfaces using RNAseZAP™ or a similar cleaning agent.
2. Depending on the nature and source of the nucleic acid sample, different preparation methods might be required. siRNA is usually provided lyophilized from the manufacturer and specified in molar quantities, whereas mRNA is normally provided in solution and specified in mass quantities. Plasmid DNA can be prepared and purified in-house using Plasmid Midi Kits (QIAGEN). All samples need to be provided at high purity and at concentrations prescribed in Table 2 (when in solution).

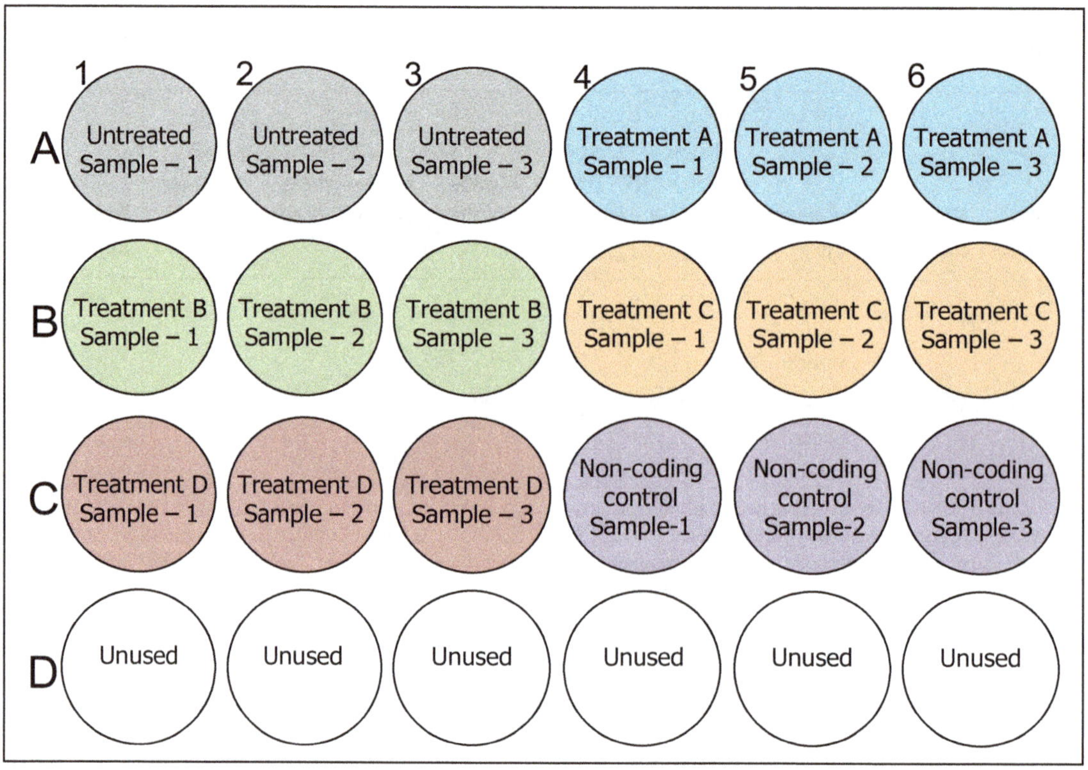

Fig. 3 Representation of a sample 24-well plate with treatments for testing the Spark Kit nanoparticles. Each condition is tested in triplicate. Refer to Table 4 for example dose amounts

3. For 2 nmol samples of lyophilized siRNA it is better to directly reconstitute in Spark Formulation Buffer 1 to minimize pipetting errors. For larger quantities, reconstitute to 20 mg/mL in nuclease-free water and aliquot. Please refer to Table 2 for more details.
4. Unused portions of Spark Formulation Buffers 1 and 2 should be refrigerated. For convenience, they can be kept with the nanoparticle mix at −80 °C.
5. To fill the wells in the Spark Cartridge, place the pipette tip just above the hole at the bottom of the well and slowly dispense the solution. Avoid bubbles during this process.
6. Store the remaining Nanoparticle Mix at −80 °C for future encapsulation.
7. To prepare larger volumes of nanoparticles, separate encapsulation of the same nucleic acid sequence can be pooled together prior to treating cells.
8. The uptake of lipid nanoparticles is enhanced in the presence of Apolipoprotein E4 (ApoE4). Some cells produce sufficient endogenous ApoE4, but others might need external ApoE4 supplementation for efficacious nanoparticle uptake. It is recommended to test treatment conditions with and without ApoE4.

9. Stock ApoE4 should be stored at −80 °C.
10. Nanoparticles and Stock ApoE4 solution can be premixed at appropriate ratios minutes prior to cell treatment to avoid extensive pipetting into individual wells.
11. For siRNA and mRNA LNPs, treatment times between 24 and 48 h are recommended. For plasmid-LNPs, treatment times between 48 and 72 h are recommended.

References

1. Cullis PR, Hope MJ (2017) Lipid nanoparticle systems for enabling gene therapies. Mol Ther 25:1467–1475. https://doi.org/10.1016/j.ymthe.2017.03.013
2. Belliveau NM, Huft J, Lin PJ et al (2012) Microfluidic synthesis of highly potent limit-size lipid nanoparticles for in vivo delivery of siRNA. Mol Ther Nucleic Acids 1:e37. https://doi.org/10.1038/mtna.2012.28
3. Lv H, Zhang S, Wang B et al (2006) Toxicity of cationic lipids and cationic polymers in gene delivery. J Control Release 114:100–109. https://doi.org/10.1016/j.jconrel.2006.04.014
4. Wu L, Nguyen LH, Zhou K et al (2015) Precise let-7 expression levels balance organ regeneration against tumor suppression. elife 4:e09431. https://doi.org/10.7554/eLife.09431
5. Yaghi NK, Wei J, Hashimoto Y et al (2017) Immune modulatory nanoparticle therapeutics for intracerebral glioma. Neuro Oncol 19:372–382. https://doi.org/10.1093/neuonc/now198
6. Ramishetti S, Landesman-Milo D, Peer D (2016) Advances in RNAi therapeutic delivery to leukocytes using lipid nanoparticles. J Drug Target 24:780–786. https://doi.org/10.3109/1061186X.2016.1172587
7. Weinstein S, Toker IA, Emmanuel R et al (2016) Harnessing RNAi-based nanomedicines for therapeutic gene silencing in B-cell malignancies. Proc Natl Acad Sci U S A 113:E16–E22. https://doi.org/10.1073/pnas.1519273113

Chapter 15

Microfluidic Assembly of Liposomes with Tunable Size and Coloading Capabilities

Jessica R. Hoffman, Ennio Tasciotti, and Roberto Molinaro

Abstract

Liposomes used for the delivery of pharmaceuticals have difficulties scaling up and reaching clinical translation as they suffer from batch-to-batch variability. Here, we describe a microfluidic approach for creating reproducible, homogenous nanoparticles with tunable characteristics. These nanoparticles of sizes ranging from 30 to 500 nm are rapidly self-assembled by controlling the flow rates of ethanol and aqueous streams. This method of microfluidic assembly allows for the efficient encapsulation of both hydrophobic and hydrophilic drugs in the lipid bilayer and particle core, respectively, either separately or in combination.

Key words Liposomes, Nanomedicine, Microfluidics, Coloading, Reproducibility, Scale up

1 Introduction

First described in 1961, liposomes, spherical nanovesicles with a lipid bilayer, have sparked a movement for the development of lipid-based nanoparticles (NP) for pharmaceutical application. However, despite a myriad of NP formulations has been proposed and developed, very few have reached clinical translation as many face problems with optimization [1]. The three traditional techniques of NP assembly, i.e., sonication, extrusion, and microfluidization, are unable to scale-up and often suffer from batch-to-batch variation, making them less viable for clinical use [2]. Microfluidics, the technology of controlling nanoliter volumes in microscale channels, offers a promising new approach to NP assembly [3]. Utilizing controlled and rapid laminar flow mixing, NPs can be molecularly self-assembled with a tunable size and consistently high homogeneity and reproducibility.

The ability to tailor NP size through the microfluidic method is advantageous for treating diseases via various administration routes. Organs allow entry to distinct sizes of NPs–particles around 150–300 nm manage to accumulate in the liver and spleen, whereas smaller NPs around 30–150 nm can accrue in the

Christoph Heuck and Niels Weinhold (eds.), *Multiple Myeloma: Methods and Protocols*, Methods in Molecular Biology, vol. 1792, https://doi.org/10.1007/978-1-4939-7865-6_15, © Springer Science+Business Media, LLC, part of Springer Nature 2018

heart and stomach [4]. Generally, particles less than 150 nm are able to cross the endothelial barrier and larger NPs undergo uptake by the mononuclear phagocytic system [4, 5]. Nonetheless, NPs of varying size are still especially beneficial with regards to cancer and inflammation as this type of tissue is often characterized by hypervascularization and leaky vasculature. NPs are able to escape circulation and penetrate diseased tissue through fenestrations ranging in size from 20 to 780 nm [6]. In particular, NPs less than 200 nm are subject to the enhanced permeability and retention effect and are able to passively invade and persist in neoplastic tissue [6]. Considering the wide application of various sized NPs, we developed a method that produces reproducible, distinctly sized particles by manipulating a few settings under microfluidic mixing.

Currently, the standard in NP surface modification and the variable most frequently adjusted to optimize the microfluidic assembly of NPs is polyethylene glycol (PEG) [7, 8, 9]. PEG was popularized as a means to shield NPs and avoid rapid clearance from the immune system. While PEG is not supposed to undergo opsonization, it has been shown that PEG can induce an immunogenic response and repeated administration can induce accelerated blood clearance [10, 11]. Furthermore, cationic lipids are another common characteristic of NPs with associated drawbacks. Cationic lipid-based NPs are frequently used to deliver DNA and RNA. However, these cationic lipids are shown to be toxic toward phagocytic cells and downregulate nitric oxide and tumor necrosis factor alpha [12]. Considering the adverse effects of PEG and cationic lipids, we avoided these materials when developing our NP formulations.

Taking into consideration the drawbacks previously mentioned, we developed unilamellar liposomes without PEG and cationic lipids that is tunable under various settings, homogenous, scalable, consistently reproducible, stable, and able to encapsulate various drugs. Utilizing the microfluidic technology of the NanoAssemblr™, various self-assembled liposomes were created by tailoring the system's temperature, total flow rate (TFR), and flow rate ratio (FRR) between aqueous and ethanol streams. Liposomal formulations were then physically characterized and tested for their ability to encapsulate hydrophilic drugs in the aqueous cores and hydrophobic drugs in the lipid bilayer. This microfluidic method allowed us to obtain liposomal formulations ranging from 30 nm to 500 nm in diameter with high homogeneity and enabled efficient encapsulation of both hydrophilic and hydrophobic drugs, either alone or in combination.

2 Materials

2.1 Liposome Assembly Materials

1. Phosphocholine-based phospholipids: 1,2-dipalmitoyl-sn-glycero-3-phosphocholine (DPPC), 1,2-dioleoyl-*sn*-glycero-3-phosphocholine (DOPC) and cholesterol (Avanti Polar Lipids).
2. 100% ethanol.
3. Deionized water.
4. 20 kDa cutoff dialysis membranes.

2.2 Micromixer

1. NanoAssemblr™ Instrument, Microfluidic Cartridges, and BT Heating Controller (Precision NanoSystems Inc.).
2. Syringes, 5 mL.
3. Syringes, 1 mL.
4. Conical tubes, 15 mL.

2.3 Characterization

1. Nanosizer ZS and Dip Cell (Malvern Instruments) for dynamic light scattering (DLS) analysis.

2.4 Drug Loading

1. Docetaxel (DTX).
2. Ammonium sulfate, 250 mM or 350 mM in DI water.
3. Ultracentrifuge.
4. Doxorubicin hydrochloride (DOX).
5. Heating block.
6. Methanol.
7. Sonicator and vortex.
8. Benchtop centrifuge.

3 Methods

Carry out all procedures at room temperature unless otherwise specified.

3.1 Assembly of NPs

1. Dissolve DPPC, DOPC, and cholesterol in 100% ethanol to create 10 mg/mL lipid stock solutions.
2. Mix the lipid components at a 4:3:3 ratio (*see* **Note 1**).
3. Wash microfluidic cartridge in the micromixer with two inlet streams of 100% ethanol and water in 5 mL syringes. Wash for a total volume of 4 mL at TFR of 12 mL/min and a FRR between water and ethanol of 3:1.
4. If the NP formulation is to be made at 45 °C, attach the NanoAssemblr™ BT Heating Controller over the chamber inlets. Otherwise, continue.

5. Load lipid–ethanol mixture into a 1 mL syringe, and place in right chamber inlet of NanoAssemblr™.
6. Load another 1 mL syringe with water and place in the left chamber inlet of the NanoAssemblr™.
7. Set FRR between the water and ethanol streams and TFR of the micromixer. We varied the FRR from 3:1 to 1:1 and TFR from 1 to 12 mL/min (*see* **Note 2**).
8. Attach waste and collection 15 mL Falcon tubes in the NanoAssemblr™.
9. Begin liposome assembly.
10. Dialyze collected liposomes overnight at 4 °C through 20 kDa dialysis membranes in 2 L of distilled water to remove residual ethanol.
11. Wash microfluidic cartridge before storing away with 100% ethanol and water using 5 mL syringes. This time, wash for a total volume of 4 mL at 12 mL/min and a FRR of 1:1.

3.2 Characterization of NPs

1. Dilute NP formulation (20uL into 1 mL water) and place in a cuvette for DLS analysis.
2. Measure NP size, polydispersity index (PDI), and zeta potential (ZP) with Nanosizer ZS. Take seven measurements, ten runs each, for each formulation. Use dip cell to measure ZP with a 60 s equilibration time (Fig. 1) (*see* **Note 3**).
3. After initial measurement, store NP formulations at 4 °C. Repeat Nanosizer ZS measurements after 1–4 weeks to ensure stability (Table 1).

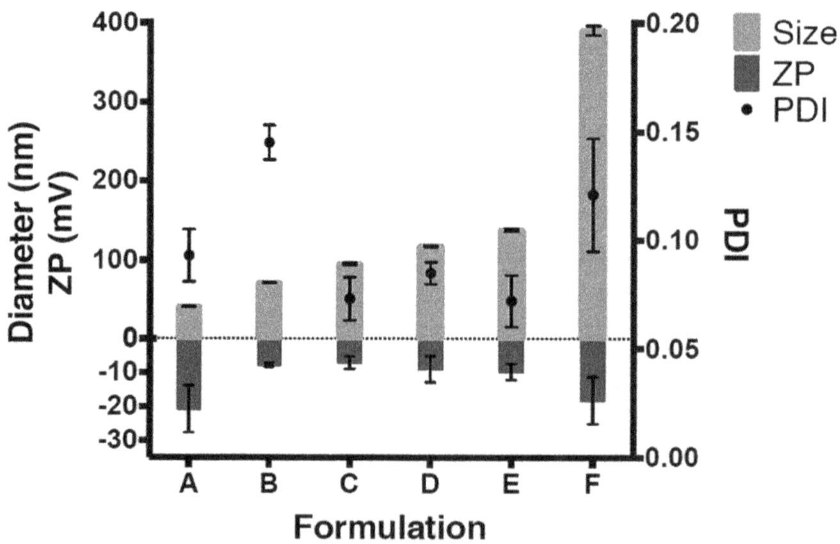

Fig. 1 Size, polydispersity index (PDI), and zeta potential (ZP) for representative Liposomal formulations

Table 1
Stability of liposomes stored under 4 °C for up to 4 weeks

Formulation		A	B	C	D	E	F
Day 0	Size (nm)	40.7 ± 0.2	71.9 ± 0.6	95.5 ± 0.9	118.0 ± 0.8	138.6 ± 2.0	390.8 ± 6.1
	PDI	0.09 ± 0.01	0.14 ± 0.01	0.07 ± 0.01	0.08 ± 0.005	0.07 ± 0.01	0.12 ± 0.02
	ZP (mV)	−20.8 ± 7.0	−7.7 ± 0.6	−7.1 ± 1.8	−9.0 ± 3.8	−9.7 ± 2.4	−18.1 ± 6.9
Week 1	Size (nm)	42.1 ± 0.3	71.0 ± 0.4	94.7 ± 0.9	123.9 ± 0.4	138.0 ± 0.9	393.4 ± 2.7
	PDI	0.09 ± 0.01	0.14 ± 0.01	0.07 ± 0.01	0.14 ± 0.01	0.10 ± 0.02	0.15 ± 0.02
	ZP (mV)	−11.9 ± 5.3	−5.9 ± 1.5	−5.2 ± 1.7	−24.9 ± 7.1	−10.4 ± 1.9	−18.1 ± 6.1
Week 4	Size (nm)	43.4 ± 0.3	70.4 ± 0.8	94.3 ± 0.8	142.2 ± 5.8	140.2 ± 1.3	393.5 ± 4.5
	PDI	0.11 ± 0.01	0.15 ± 0.01	0.06 ± 0.02	0.29 ± 0.02	0.11 ± 0.03	0.12 ± 0.04
	ZP (mV)	−11.1 ± 4.1	−6.7 ± 1.2	−4.9 ± 1.6	−24.8 ± 10.6	−17.2 ± 4.3	−18.6 ± 5.5

3.3 Drug Loading

Docetaxel (DTX) and doxorubicin (DOX) were used as proof-of-principle hydrophobic and hydrophilic drug molecules, respectively. Both drugs were loaded separately and in combination.

1. To create drug-loaded liposomes, increase the amount of lipids per formulation to 27 mM, keeping the same 4:3:3 ratio as before (*see* **Note 4**).
2. To load DTX in the NP bilayer, dissolve 10 mol% of DTX (mol drug:mol lipid) in the ethanol–lipid mixture prior to NanoAssemblr™ mixing.
3. DOX was remotely loaded in the aqueous core of liposomes using an ammonium sulfate gradient. Load either 250–350 mM ammonium sulfate into the aqueous syringe. We compared liposomes assembled through thin-layer evaporation (TLE) method and microfluidic mixing with 250–350 mM ammonium sulfate (*see* **Note 5**). We observed the greatest encapsulation efficiency (EE%) with microfluidic assembled NPs using 350 mM ammonium sulfate (Table 2).
4. Ultracentrifuge formulation at 36,000 × *g* for 1 h at 4 °C to remove excess ammonium sulfate.
5. Remove supernatant and resuspend pellet in 2 mg/mL of DOX and incubate on a heating block for 2 h at 45 °C.
6. Ultracentrifuge using the previous settings to remove not-encapsulated DOX. Remove the supernatant and resuspend pellet in 1 mL methanol for EE analysis.
7. Sonicate and vortex until the pellet is broken up (about 1 h) (*see* **Note 6**).

Table 2
Encapsulation efficiency, size, and polydispersity index (PDI) of DOX-loaded liposomes assembled through thin-layer evaporation (TLE) and microfluidic mixing (MM) with 250 mM or 250 mM of ammonium sulfate

FRR	TFR	Method	EE %	Size (nm)	PDI
2:1	1	TLE	58.9%	139.5 ± 2.2	0.444 ± 0.011
		MM, 250 mM	54.9%	134.0 ± 1.5	0.111 ± 0.016
		MM, 350 mM	83.9%	137.1 ± 1.2	0.219 ± 0.007
2:1	9	TLE	71.1%	88.1 ± 0.9	0.167 ± 0.014
		MM, 250 mM	70.1%	92.8 ± 1.2	0.080 ± 0.011
		MM, 350 mM	87.5%	83.1 ± 0.5	0.092 ± 0.011
3:1	12	TLE	69.2%	105.8 ± 1.1	0.226 ± 0.010
		MM, 250 mM	33.3%	76.9 ± 0.8	0.142 ± 0.010
		MM, 350 mM	30.5%	74.6 ± 0.6	0.145 ± 0.011

Only the formulations that resulted stable after the synthesis process are reported

Table 3
Encapsulation efficiency, size, and polydispersity index (PDI) of DTX-loaded liposomes assembled through thin-layer evaporation (TLE) and microfluidic mixing (MM). Only the formulations that resulted stable after the synthesis process are reported

FRR	TFR	EE %	Size (nm)	PDI
TLE	–	35%	158	0.18
2:1	1	12.3%	70	0.20
2:1	9	33.3%	165	0.44
3:1	12	6.4%	50	0.11

8. Filter sample for 5 min at 20,000 × g in 0.45 μm Eppendorf filter.
9. Collect filtered sample and use HPLC to determine DTX encapsulation at its typical wavelength (227 nm). Measure DOX EE through spectrofluorimetric analysis at the excitation and emission wavelengths of DOX, i.e., 480–560 nm, respectively (Table 3).
10. Liposomes loaded with DTX and DOX were also generated and encapsulation efficiency of both drugs was determined (Table 4).

Table 4
Encapsulation efficiency of DTX and DOX-loaded Liposomes

FRR	TFR	DTX EE %	DOX EE%	Size (nm)	PDI
2:1	1	14.7	70	70.2	0.20
2:1	9	29	68	117.5	0.25

Table 5
Amount of lipids per empty liposomal formulations

FRR	DPPC (mg)	CHOL (mg)	DOPC (mg)	Lipid Concentration (μmol)
3:1	1.98	0.78	1.59	6.75
2:1	2.64	1.04	2.12	9.00
3:2	3.17	1.25	2.55	10.80
1:1	3.96	1.57	3.18	13.50

4 Notes

1. All lipid mixtures of DPPC, cholesterol and DOPC were made at a 4:3:3 molar ratio. For empty formulations, the amounts of lipids varied between FRR (Table 5).
2. The size of the Liposomes was controlled primarily by the FRR and secondarily by the TFR. Size increases with a decreasing FRR and TFR. The greatest homogeneity ($PDI < 0.1$) was observed in formulations with a FRR of 2:1.
3. Each possible combination of NP was created from varying TFR (1, 3, 6, 9, and 12 mL/min), FRR (1:1, 3:2, 2:1, and 1:1), and temperature (room temperature or 45 °C) (Table 6). Six representative NP formulations were chosen as they exhibited a wide range of sizes with high homogeneity (Table 7).
4. We found the greatest success with loading hydrophobic and hydrophilic drugs by increasing the lipid amount to 27 mM. The same 4:3:3 ratio was kept between lipids with 8.16 mg DPPC, 3.22 mg cholesterol, and 6.55 mg DOPC dissolved in 100% ethanol per formulation.
5. Thin-layer evaporation technique was used to produce liposomes as control. Briefly, DPPC, DOPC, and cholesterol were dissolved in chloroform–methanol (3:1 v/v) at 4:3:3 molar ratio. The organic solvent has been evaporated under vacuum

Table 6
Size, PDI, and zeta potential (ZP) of liposomes assembled under various microfluidic mixing settings

		Room Temperature			45 °C		
FRR	**TFR**	**Size**	**PDI**	**ZP**	**Size**	**PDI**	**ZP**
3:1	1	84.2 ± 0.6	0.161 ± 0.012	−11.4 ± 0.9	69.0 ± 0.7	0.18 ± 0.005	−17.4 ± 5.8
	3	71.9 ± 0.6	0.145 ± 0.008	−7.7 ± 0.6	54.9 ± 0.5	0.19 ± 0.015	−13.4 ± 1.7
	6	48.6 ± 0.4	0.143 ± 0.004	−11.6 ± 3.4	34.7 ± 0.3	0.15 ± 0.013	−17.5 ± 2.4
	9	39.1 ± 0.3	0.135 ± 0.025	−19.7 ± 4.9	34.8 ± 0.2	0.15 ± 0.016	−13.1 ± 2.1
	12	40.7 ± 0.2	0.093 ± 0.012	−20.8 ± 7.0	37.7 ± 0.1	0.23 ± 0.027	−3.7 ± 2.4
2:1	1	138.6 ± 2.0	0.072 ± 0.012	−9.7 ± 2.4	118.0 ± 0.1	0.13 ± 0.063	−12.2 ± 1.2
	3	105.6 ± 0.6	0.082 ± 0.014	−7.0 ± 1.3	78.3 ± 0.8	0.05 ± 0.021	−6.7 ± 1.3
	6	89.5 ± 0.4	0.070 ± 0.013	−7.8 ± 3.4	73.4 ± 0.5	0.06 ± 0.007	−12.8 ± 1.6
	9	95.5 ± 0.9	0.073 ± 0.010	−7.1 ± 1.8	85.6 ± 0.5	0.07 ± 0.018	−5.2 ± 1.8
	12	68.2 ± 0.1	0.058 ± 0.013	−9.4 ± 3.2	67.8 ± 0.3	0.05 ± 0.013	−7.5 ± 1.1
3:2	1	144.8 ± 0.9	0.107 ± 0.019	−5.8 ± 2.0	129.0 ± 0.8	0.09 ± 0.017	−10.8 ± 2.1
	3	131.2 ± 1.5	0.116 ± 0.013	−8.2 ± 2.2	99.2 ± 0.6	0.10 ± 0.020	−9.4 ± 3.0
	6	129.8 ± 1.7	0.160 ± 0.018	−8.6 ± 2.3	103.9 ± 1.3	0.08 ± 0.009	−6.7 ± 2.1
	9	121.4 ± 1.0	0.184 ± 0.006	−7.8 ± 2.3	89.55 ± 1.2	0.08 ± 0.014	−6.1 ± 1.4
	12	115.2 ± 1.1	0.229 ± 0.014	−9.6 ± 2.4	93.1 ± 0.7	0.10 ± 0.069	−12.6 ± 3.5
1:1	1	390.8 ± 6.1	0.121 ± 0.026	−18.1 ± 6.9	351.6 ± 1.7	0.15 ± 0.024	−17.9 ± 3.1
	3	360.1 ± 2.6	0.171 ± 0.020	−15.6 ± 3.5	486.2 ± 7.1	0.32 ± 0.033	−18.2 ± 1.8
	6	608.6 ± 10.9	0.261 ± 0.014	−14.6 ± 4.2	341.1 ± 4.2	0.12 ± 0.011	−16.4 ± 1.7
	9	389.8 ± 5.6	0.121 ± 0.027	−14.3 ± 6.2	563.7 ± 6.1	0.26 ± 0.014	−16.1 ± 1.7
	12	423.4 ± 6.1	0.151 ± 0.041	−15.0 ± 2.7	414.0 ± 6.6	0.10 ± 0.033	−18.0 ± 1.8

Table 7
Representative liposomal formulations

Formulation	FRR	TFR	Temp (°C)
A	3:1	12	23
B	3:1	3	23
C	2:1	9	23
D	2:1	1	45
E	2:1	1	23
F	1:1	1	23

using a rotary evaporator (BUCHI Labortechnik AG, Flawil, Switzerland). The obtained film was then hydrated with distilled water to obtain a lipid concentration of 27 mM. Unilamellar liposomes were then obtained through extrusion using 200 nm pore cellulose acetate membranes (Whatman, Schleicher & Schuell) at 45 °C. DOX was encapsulated using the remote loading protocol after lipid film hydration with ammonium sulfate (250 mM), ultracentrifugation at 36,000 × *g* for 1 h at 4 °C to remove excess ammonium sulfate, and incubation with 2 mg/mL of DOX on a heating block for 2 h at 45 °C. For DTX loading, the drug (10 mol% mol drug:mol lipid) was dissolved in the chloroform–methanol mixture.

6. Liposomes are not particularly soluble in methanol. Avoid using a pipette to transfer the formulation unnecessarily.

Acknowledgments

This work was supported by grants RF-2010-2318372 and RF-2010-2305526 from the Italian Ministry of Health, William Randolph Hearst Foundation, The Regenerative Medicine Program Cullen Trust for Health Care (Project ID: 18130014), Brown Foundation (Project ID:18130011), the Hearst Foundation (Project ID: 18130017), the NIH/NCI and the Office of Research on Women's Health (Grant # 1R56CA213859), and Cancer Prevention and Research Institute of Texas (Project ID: RP170466) to E.T. The authors acknowledge the George J. and Angelina P. Kostas Charitable Foundation and CARIPARO Foundation Ricerca Pediatrica 2016–2018 Grant.

References

1. Shi J, Xiao Z, Kamaly N, Farokhzad OC (2011) Self-assembled targeted nanoparticles: evolution of technologies and bench to bedside translation. Acc Chem Res 44(10):1123–1134. https://doi.org/10.1021/ar200054n
2. Belliveau NM et al (2012) Microfluidic synthesis of highly potent limit-size lipid nanoparticles for in vivo delivery of siRNA. Mol Ther Nucleic Acids 1:e37. https://doi.org/10.1038/mtna.2012.28
3. Valencia PM, Pridgen EM, Rhee M, Langer R, Farokhzad OC, Karnik R (2013) Microfluidic platform for combinatorial synthesis and optimization of targeted nanoparticles for cancer therapy. ACS Nano 7(12):10671–10680. https://doi.org/10.1021/nn403370e
4. Gaumet M, Vargas A, Gurny R, Delie F (2008) Nanoparticles for drug delivery: the need for precision in reporting particle size parameters. Eur J Pharm Biopharm 69(1):1–9. https://doi.org/10.1016/j.ejpb.2007.08.001
5. Maeda H, Wu J, Sawa T, Matsumura Y, Hori K (2000) Tumor vascular permeability and the EPR effect in macromolecular therapeutics: a review. J Control Release 65(1–2):271–284. https://doi.org/10.1016/S0168-3659(99)00248-5
6. He C, Hu Y, Yin L, Tang C, Yin C (2010) Effects of particle size and surface charge on cellular uptake and biodistribution of polymeric nanoparticles. Biomaterials 31(13):3657–3666. https://doi.org/10.1016/j.biomaterials.2010.01.065
7. Knop K, Hoogenboom R, Fischer D, Schubert US (2010) Poly(ethylene glycol) in drug delivery: pros and cons as well as potential alternatives. ChemInform 42:3. https://doi.org/10.1002/chin.201103264

8. Walsh C et al (2014) Microfluidic-based manufacture of siRNA-lipid nanoparticles for therapeutic applications. Methods Mol Biol 1141:109–120. https://doi.org/10.1007/978-1-4939-0363-4_6
9. Zhigaltsev IV et al (2016) Production of limit size nanoliposomal systems with potential utility as ultra-small drug delivery agents. J Liposome Res 26(2):96–102. https://doi.org/10.3109/08982104.2015.1025411
10. Corbo C, Molinaro R, Parodi A, Toledano-Furman NE, Salvatore F, Tasciotti E (2016) The impact of nanoparticle protein corona on cytotoxicity, immunotoxicity and target drug delivery. Nanomedicine 11(1):81–100. https://doi.org/10.2217/nnm.15.188
11. Wolfram J et al (2014) The nano-plasma interface: implications of the protein corona. Colloids Surf B: Biointerfaces 124:17–24. https://doi.org/10.1016/j.colsurfb.2014.02.035
12. Filion MC, Phillips NC (1997) Toxicity and immunomodulatory activity of liposomal vectors formulated with cationic lipids toward immune effector cells. Biochim Biophys Acta Biomembr 1329(2):345–356. https://doi.org/10.1016/S0005-2736(97)00126-0

Retraction Note to: EuroFlow-Based Next-Generation Flow Cytometry for Detection of Circulating Tumor Cells and Minimal Residual Disease in Multiple Myeloma

Leire Burgos and Bruno Paiva

Retraction Note to:
Chapter "EuroFlow-Based Next-Generation Flow Cytometry for Detection of Circulating Tumor Cells and Minimal Residual Disease in Multiple Myeloma" in: Christoph Heuck and Niels Weinhold (eds.), *Multiple Myeloma: Methods and Protocols*, Methods in Molecular Biology, vol. 1792, https://doi.org/10.1007/978-1-4939-7865-6_2

The chapter published in the book 'Multiple Myeloma', pages 15-34, https://doi.org/10.1007/978-1-4939-7865-6_2 has been retracted due to the following reasons:

- The authors have used the EuroFlow methods for many years (EuroFlow membership since 2013) and have built extensive experience with the application of these methods, they did not contribute to the design and standardization of the EuroFlow methods. Other members of the EuroFlow consortium have developed and standardized the methods and tools over a period of more than 6 years (2006-2012). These EuroFlow members have not been informed about the writing of the book chapter and have not been acknowledged as the original designers of the presented methods.
- The authors used EuroFlow proprietary information and figures without asking permission and without appropriate reference to the relevant EuroFlow publications or EuroFlow website documents.

The authors deeply regret the inconvenience caused by the retraction.

The retracted online version of this chapter can be found at https://doi.org/10.1007/978-1-4939-7865-6_2

Christoph Heuck and Niels Weinhold (eds.), *Multiple Myeloma: Methods and Protocols*, Methods in Molecular Biology, vol. 1792, https://doi.org/10.1007/978-1-4939-7865-6_16, © Springer Science+Business Media, LLC, part of Springer Nature 2018

Correction to: Multiple Myeloma

Christoph Heuck and Niels Weinhold

Correction to:
Christoph Heuck and Niels Weinhold (eds.), *Multiple Myeloma: Methods and Protocols*, Methods in Molecular Biology, vol. 1792, https://doi.org/10.1007/978-1-4939-7865-6

In Chapter 4, the author's name Homer Adams III has been modified to Adams HC 3rd, as requested by him.

In Chapter 13 (page no. 186), the text in bold font in the below sentence has been revised to the following.

Section: **3.8 (Bisulfite Conversion)**

2. Meanwhile, prepare the bisulfite conversion (CT) reagent by **mixing 210 μL of ultrapure water and 750 μL of M-dilution buffer** to the content of CT-reagents per vial (*see* **Note 7**).

Has been replaced with

2. Meanwhile, prepare the bisulfite conversion (CT) reagent by **mixing 210 μL of Mdilution buffer and 750 μL of ultrapure water** to the content of CT-reagents per vial (*see* **Note 7**).

The updated online versions of these chapters can be found at
https://doi.org/10.1007/978-1-4939-7865-6_4
https://doi.org/10.1007/978-1-4939-7865-6_13

Christoph Heuck and Niels Weinhold (eds.), *Multiple Myeloma: Methods and Protocols*, Methods in Molecular Biology, vol. 1792, https://doi.org/10.1007/978-1-4939-7865-6_17, © Springer Science+Business Media, LLC, part of Springer Nature 2020

Index

B

Barcoding 48, 50, 53, 187
Bioinformatics 148, 149, 158
Bisulfite conversion 180, 186, 187
Bone marrow (BM) 1, 17, 23, 25, 26, 28, 29, 31, 32, 36, 38, 39, 47–49, 55–57, 64, 77, 97, 119, 130, 157, 160, 180, 195

C

Cancer cytogenetics 55
Cell-free DNA (cfDNA) 129–136, 139, 142, 143
Circulating cell-free nucleic acids 131, 133
Circulating tumor cells (CTC) 15
Circulating tumor DNA (ctDNA) 129–144
CIg/DNA 36
Clinical application 97, 157
Coloading 205
Cytometry by Time-of-Flight (CyTOF) 47–54
Cytoplasmic immunoglobulin (CIg) 35–44

D

Data mining 158
DNA Index (DI) 35, 42
DNA methylation 167, 168, 179, 180, 186
DNA probes 55–58, 61–63
Droplet digital PCR (ddPCR) 130–133, 135–140, 143, 144, 148–152

E

Encapsulation 193, 196, 202, 206, 209–211
EuroFlow 15, 21

F

Flow cytometry 1, 15–33, 35, 47, 201
Fluorescence in situ hybridization (FISH) 55–64, 71, 73

G

GenomicScape 158–163
β-Glucosyl transferase 169

H

HpaII 167–176
5 Hydroxymethycytosine 168, 169

I

Immunoglobulin (IG) 2, 5–6, 16, 35, 56, 71
Immunophenotyping 22, 26, 28, 30, 47, 48

K

Kappa and lambda 2, 16, 39, 41, 42, 56, 59, 65

L

Library preparation 103, 105–109, 113, 118, 120, 126, 180
Lipid nanoparticle (LNP) 193–203
Liposomes 205–213
Liquid biopsy 129
Low input 97, 180

M

Mass cytometry 47, 48
Messenger RNA (mRNA) 195–198, 201
5 Methylcytosine 167
Microarrays 97, 98, 157–160
Microfluidics 193, 205, 210, 212
Minimal residual disease (MRD) 1, 10, 15
Molecular heterogeneity 157
MspI 168, 169, 171, 172, 180–182
Multiple myeloma (MM) 1, 15, 36, 47, 55, 71, 97, 117, 130, 147, 157, 167, 180
MYC 71–93

N

Nanomedicine 205
Next generation flow (NGF) 15
Next-generation sequencing (NGS) 1, 117, 126, 129–131, 147, 180

P

Peripheral blood (PB) 1, 16–19, 23, 26, 38, 55, 64, 77, 130, 131, 133, 139

Christoph Heuck and Niels Weinhold (eds.), *Multiple Myeloma: Methods and Protocols*, Methods in Molecular Biology, vol. 1792,
https://doi.org/10.1007/978-1-4939-7865-6,

Peripheral blood plasma 130, 139
Plasmid 68, 196–198, 201, 203

Q

qASO-PCR 1–12

R

Rearrangements 2, 5–6, 55, 72, 73, 76, 180
Reduced representation bisulfite
sequencing (RRBS) 179, 181
Reproducibility 17, 22, 205
RNA-sequencing 97–113, 148
RNAi 193

S

Scale-up 99, 205
Sequencing 1, 2, 5, 6, 12, 71, 97, 117–126, 129, 147–155, 168, 179–190
Single-cell 16, 32, 47, 147
Size selection 81–82, 107, 180, 185
Small interfering RNA (siRNA) 195–203
Smart Tube 47–49, 51
Somatic mutations 72, 119, 125, 126
Standard diagnostic workflow 117

T

Targeted sequencing panel 117, 153
Transfection 193, 196
Translocations 55, 56, 71

W

Whole exome sequencing (WES) 71–93, 117, 118, 129

www.ingramcontent.com/pod-product-compliance
Lightning Source LLC
Chambersburg PA
CBHW080735150926
51501CB00005B/166
* 9 7 8 1 4 9 3 9 7 8 6 4 9 *